The Truth About
Carpal Tunnel Syndrome

The Truth About
Carpal Tunnel Syndrome

Finding Answers, Getting Well

Jill Gambaro

ROWMAN & LITTLEFIELD
Lanham • Boulder • New York • Toronto • Plymouth, UK

Published by Rowman & Littlefield
4501 Forbes Boulevard, Suite 200, Lanham, Maryland 20706
www.rowman.com

10 Thornbury Road, Plymouth PL6 7PP, United Kingdom

British Library Cataloguing in Publication Information Available

Library of Congress Cataloging-in-Publication Data

Gambaro, Jill, 1959-
The truth about carpal tunnel syndrome : finding answers, getting well / Jill Gambaro.
pages cm
Includes bibliographical references and index.
ISBN 978-1-4422-2579-4 (cloth : alk. paper) -- ISBN 978-1-4422-2580-0 (electronic)
1. Carpal tunnel syndrome. 2. Carpal tunnel syndrome--Treatment. 3. Overuse injuries--Miscellanea. I. Title.
RC422.C26G36 2014
616.85'6--dc23
2013051337

Printed in the United States of America

To anyone who has ever tried to express themselves with their hands.

Contents

Introduction

This book was difficult to write, not least because of my disabilities. Many I interviewed were cautious about what they said and wanted to approve any quotes I attributed to them. Many disagreed with others' comments. Some, including doctors, lawyers, risk managers, and insurance researchers, wouldn't even talk to me. Several people suggested that I coauthor the book with an MD, but I knew that wouldn't allow me to write the book I felt was needed. Not everyone will agree with what I say. At least I've sparked a conversation—likely a very heated one.

Not everyone agreed with the need for a book from the patient's perspective. Those of us who contract repetitive strain injuries (RSIs) must learn to live with them. We have to find a way to understand them that allows us to begin to undo the damage that's been done. Frankly, we care less about definitive science than about our quality of life. When you are a patient suffering with a "medical mystery," you face not only the devastation of a catastrophic illness but also the tough road of fighting for a quality of care that does not exist, no matter what the professionals tell you. Those who treat RSIs either tell you with absolute confidence that they can fix the problem or say that there's no medical evidence to support your symptoms. Both stances are true as well as false.

It is very frustrating, when you are not a scientist and have not been trained in medicine, to be expected to make life-altering decisions. I couldn't find a doctor to advise me about whether or not to have back surgery. No one wanted to assume the liability.

I am not a doctor; I'm a writer and filmmaker. I have no training in health care. There are others more qualified to write about the science of RSIs, but they risk their jobs by doing so. No one can fire me; I've already lost my job. Nothing I say in this book should be taken as medical advice. Nothing I say in this book should be taken for the whole truth. No one knows the whole truth about RSIs right now, which is why so many still contract them.

Everything about RSIs is complex: their physiology, politics, and legal, economic, and sociological issues. The real stakeholders—patients, employers, and doctors—aren't the ones in charge. Plenty claim to understand what causes them. Plenty show evidence backing up their point of view. Their certainty is necessary for them to proceed along their line of scientific inquiry, and we need their definitiveness, even if it isn't the whole truth. As I write this, I'm sitting in a coffee shop across from a woman wearing a wrist brace. Last night I went to a dinner party and met an Olympic athlete who had unsuccessful carpal tunnel surgery. When I went to my local Social Security office to tell them I was writing the book, the stoic clerks allowed wry smiles to slip onto their faces. Every one of us is a stakeholder in RSIs.

I have written this book in an attempt to bridge the gap between patients and doctors, researchers and clinicians, workers and employers, politicians and policy makers, scientists and lawyers. I'm striving to change average people's understanding of RSIs so that they don't rely on the government, their doctors, or their employers. There's a disconnect between what the medical establishment is willing to endorse and what a patient is willing to live with. This is the real crux of health-care reform.

I have not been cured of my RSIs; I have only learned to manage them. I have to remain vigilant about the types of tasks I do and how often, how much exercise I get, and how much sitting and standing and walking I do. Constantly. I'm always looking for ways to be able to do more. If I stop exercising or sit too long or type too much, I get a flare-up. Pain comes crashing down on me again, along with fear and anxiety.

We may not all be world-renowned concert pianists or surgeons, but we all rely heavily on the use of our hands. You can work without your legs or your sight but not without your hands. They are a very intimate part of us, and to lose use of them affects our ability to express ourselves and to care for our loved ones and ourselves.

Many thanks to all the brave people who did agree to be quoted in these pages—specifically, to Dr. George Piligian, Dr. James D. Collins, Dr. Marian Garfinkel, Greg Dempster, Bonnie Prestridge, and Jonathan Bailin, who helped shape the book and reviewed much of the material. Also, thanks to the Los Angeles Repetitive Strain Injury Support Group and to all the RSI sufferers I've met over the years. Your stories helped me go on. Finally, thank you to my personal team, all of whom acted as my sounding board and support system: my publisher, Suzanne Staszak-Silva; my agent, Rich Henshaw; and Susanna Bond, Elaine Dodd, Carver Irish, Nancy Bliven, Taniya Hossain, Joe Goshert, Alex Goshert-Hossain, and Jennifer Martin. Lastly, thanks to Fidel, who curled up beside me during much of the writing.

I used Dragon voice-recognition software for Mac to write the book. It's less accurate than Dragon for PC that I used successfully for years. I still had to edit by hand with the Mac version. I would have been able to do a good deal of the editing using voice recognition with Dragon for PC.

.

Chapter One

I Woke Up One Morning to Find My Life Had Fallen Apart

It all started with a strange sensation in my left palm—not what I would call pain, just a tingling. It was as if I had slept on my hand or a bee had somehow became trapped inside, its venom pulling my thumb and pinky together. But when I looked at my hand, it looked perfectly normal. I kept stretching it open and rubbing my palm, trying to figure out what was causing the strange sensation. Had I somehow compressed my hand under the pillow during the night? Unlike when a limb has fallen asleep, this didn't go away. After a few days, I mentioned it to a friend who is a medical illustrator. She said, "That's not your hand. That's your neck."

I grew up in an Italian neighborhood on the east side of Detroit. Three generations of Gambaros lived there, not to mention countless aunts, uncles, and cousins. Everyone knew me before I knew them: the old man in the dime store who'd let me slide if I was a few pennies short, the burly butcher who always gave me a few slices of salami to nibble on while I waited, the nice ladies at the bakery who slipped me a few powdered-sugar puffs called "angel wings" whenever my mom sent me in for bread. "You're Mario's granddaughter, aren't you?"

We didn't have much in the way of money, but we had our integrity, and my grandfather believed that made us rich. At the age of nineteen, he had sailed alone from a small village in Italy; he didn't speak a word of English when he arrived in the United States but made his way through a reputation for hard work. He entered the construction trade, helped build a union, and played bocce, the Italian lawn game, on Sundays at Buddy's Pizzeria. His legacy, more than anything else, has helped me make my way in the world. I was born with his wandering heart and wanted to see what lay beyond the old neighborhood. By the time I was twenty-one, I, too, had set off from home.

1

In the years since, I have led an adventurous life. I've lived in five states, been to twice as many countries, and written about them all. It's hard to make a living as a writer; I've had to pay my dues. I picked up temporary jobs here and there to keep money coming in. If I were a man, I'd be considered a jack-of-all-trades, but I'm a woman and a fast typist, so I found work in offices as a temporary secretary.

Being a temp was great: put in eight hours and get a check at the end of the day. To stay out of office politics and maintain the flexibility to travel, I moved around a lot. Usually I worked only a few days a week, or a few weeks a month, or a few months in a row before taking time off to write or, later, to make a film. Just like my grandfather, I had built a reputation for hard work and dependability. A long list of regular clients kept me busy.

Having just cracked the print world writing for newspapers and magazines, I was flush with the excitement of publishing every month. I was also enjoying a new romantic relationship and giddy with love. While blissfully occupied, I somehow wound up working forty hours a week for three different law firms over a nine-month stretch for the first time in at least a dozen years. I came in every morning, donned the headphones, and zoned out as my fingers flew. I didn't realize I was typing 125 words a minute, seven hours a day, five days a week. And the more work I did, the more work they gave me. What started in my hands quickly spread to the middle of my back. Every time I reached—for a stapler, the phone, or a brush—it hurt. You have no idea how often you reach for something during the day until you feel searing pain each time you do.

My first thought was to see a chiropractor, but like so many Americans, I had no health insurance. While I was saving the money for an office visit, the pain that started in my hand spread into the middle of my back, up into my neck, and across my shoulders. The chiropractor seemed to think my pain was routine enough. Discounting his usual fee, he told me one session a week for four weeks should clear it up. But it didn't. Instead, the pain grew worse. Little by little, more and more movements shot painful flames throughout my upper body until I couldn't reach outward, forward, above my head, or below my waist without crying out. I couldn't wash my hair, prepare a meal, open a door, or wipe myself. I bought a lumbar roll for my chair at work and a neck roll for the car. I used a heating pad, pulled all my desk tools close to me, and kept my body as still as possible. Nothing helped. In two short months, even with treatment, my shoulders froze, and I could barely move my arms, hands, or fingers at all. Clearly I couldn't work anymore.

I didn't want to admit that work was the cause; yet the evidence mounted. The pain was much less on Sunday night than on Wednesday morning. When my bosses asked me what was wrong, I blamed my pain on other things. They were just as happy to deny the problem as I was. One morning, I got a call from a boss on his way into work. He started dictating a letter to me over the phone. Since I couldn't hold the phone to my ear with my shoulder anymore, I put him on speakerphone. But he was on his cell, going through a dead spot, and I couldn't hear a thing. "What? Say that again?" Frustrated and angry, he asked, "Didn't you just come back from the chiropractor?" We all knew something was wrong, but we all ignored the proverbial elephant in the room.

I thought I wouldn't qualify for workers' compensation because I was a temp. Under the law, however, I was an employee of the firms where I was temping because I worked in their offices, on their equipment, during hours they set. Still, I wasn't sure my bosses had reported me to their insurance carriers. If they hadn't, my claim would get them into trouble. I didn't want to do that. After all, it wasn't as if they had tried to hurt me. In their defense, none of them knew how much I did on my other jobs or the extent to which my workload had increased overall. And none of them knew the computer was the problem.

As a freelancer, I relied on my reputation in the community, and over the years I had built a sterling one. In the legal field, everyone knows exactly what is and is not legal. I knew if I filed a claim, word would get out, and I would lose my livelihood. I knew if I still had to work for the lawyers I had filed a claim against, they would make my life miserable, regardless of how illegal that would be. They'd know how to get around the law. Later, I found my fears justified.

My only option was to quit typing. It was the middle of December, so I decided after the first of the year that I would look for another job—one in which I didn't have to type so much. But everything I knew about carpal tunnel syndrome was wrong. Word in the lunchroom was that you have surgery, recover for a few short weeks, and go back to work. Without health insurance, I hoped my hands would last long enough so that I could make the career move and dodge the surgical bill and the damaging claim. I never made it that far.

I thought my arms had swelled but never realized that lesions were scarring my connective tissue. My hands were so far gone that I couldn't move my fingers. When they did move, gobbledygook came out. I was not only a fast typist; I was a very accurate one. I made two or three typical errors, but that was all. Suddenly, weird things began appearing on my computer screen, like "t-h-e-r-e" instead of "t-h-e-i-r." Where did that come from? Those aren't even similar keystrokes. I thought one thing, and something else entirely appeared. Routine, complex muscle movements were going completely haywire. Because my injury, at that time, was only in my upper body, I only noticed that my hands were out of control. I didn't yet realize that this was neurological damage—very serious neurological damage.

When my month of sessions had elapsed, my chiropractor broke the bad news: I needed more treatment. I had no way to pay for it. I mentioned this to all my employers, hoping we could finally talk about that elephant. After all, they knew the status of their workers' compensation insurance; they knew that I would qualify. In retrospect, I understand that they were just as jolted by the situation as I was. For a small business with only one or two employees, a claim like mine could spell financial ruin. I just had to get past the holidays and into January, when companies begin hiring again. I just had to keep right on working.

My shoulders forced the decision on me one Thursday in the middle of January. Unfortunately, when I got to the office, I found a long typing assignment waiting for me. I remember thinking, Boy, if I can just make it to the weekend . . . I typed slower. It wasn't enough. I waited for my lunch hour. By two o'clock, my shoulders were throbbing, so I fashioned makeshift ice packs and balanced them on either side of my neck. I kept sneaking into the conference room every fifteen minutes to lie on the floor just so I could go on. By four o'clock, my knuckles had locked, and my fingers would only move up and down from the palm. My neck burned and buzzed unbearably. My shoulders contracted into a charley horse that took two years to relax. My entire upper body had seized into one continual throe. To this day, I can't believe it never occurred to me simply to stop typing.

I have since noticed that those of us who contract RSIs tend to be type A personalities. While on the board of directors of the Los Angeles Repetitive Strain Injury Support Group, I took the initial inquiry calls. I remember one woman in particular who told me how the small business she was working for had to keep laying off workers to survive, so that by the time she couldn't work anymore, she was the secretary, bookkeeper, receptionist, stock boy, and relocation coordinator. With the economy as bad as it's been since 2008, those lucky enough to have a job are often asked to double up on duties.

On Friday morning, the day after my body seized, I awoke to find that my entire life had fallen apart. I don't know how I drove my stick shift that morning. As it was, I staggered into my chiropractor's office hunched over like a ninety-year-old woman. The entire examination went by as if in a dream—the X-rays, the neck brace, and then the dreadful news: "I'm taking you off work." When my chiropractor brought in the black Velcro collar, I sobbed. Whenever I'd seen people wearing them in the past, I always thought they were faking it for big bucks. "Do I have to wear that in public?" Despite how they fussed over me and the look in their eyes, I still refused to believe it was that bad.

I didn't even know what questions to ask. As for a diagnosis, I never really got one. I only heard my chiropractor say that I would be off work for about a month. I thought he was exaggerating. I thought I just had a backache. Little did I know, he was practicing psychology as well as chiropractic. He kept saying, "It's not the worst I've ever seen."

I finally got the nerve to ask, "What is the worst you've ever seen?"

"On a scale of one to ten, ten being the worst case I've ever seen?"

I nodded.

"A nine."

Still, I didn't believe him. He set up a treatment protocol, scheduled me for four visits a week, and sent me home. I barely heard a word he said. My whole world had come to a standstill. My mind tried to race through the pain. If you can't make good decisions when you're emotional, you really can't make them when you're in pain. I suddenly faced a slew of problems that I had to navigate on my own. I needed an attorney, and I needed one fast.

Despite all my years working within the legal community, I knew nothing about workers' compensation—other than the conventional wisdom that anyone who files a claim is taking. I called a few professional acquaintances and got a few recommendations—as well as a lot of cold shoulders. The first referral refused to take the case because he considered my employers his colleagues. Others said, "You're case is too complicated. I can't make any money off of that." To make matters worse, the more calls I made, the more frantic I became, and the more my neck burned. Nervous tension, you see, excites your neurological system and actually increases RSI pain.

I finally found a lawyer who agreed to see me. As I sat in his office, he looked at me like I had become paralyzed and he was next. He was the first person other than a doctor, employer, or friend to comment on my condition. It was then that I realized how serious my injury was. He said I didn't have to tell my employers that I was filing the claim; they would find out soon enough. But I wasn't raised that way. It seemed common courtesy to tell them myself. Besides, they couldn't fire me or discriminate against me because of it. One of them told me to rest up and let him know when I would be able to return to work. He assured me my job would be waiting for me. The other two hit the ceiling. One claimed that because I'd never showed up that day, I'd abandoned my job. The other denied that I worked there at all. In a few days, both sent me threatening letters. I was not concerned; I knew they were breaking the law and that justice would be served. It never was.

My lawyer made an appointment for me to see an MD because the California workers' compensation system, at the time, did not consider chiropractors qualified to run point on a medical case. But the orthopedic surgeon was booked for six weeks.

Over the next few days, I could do none of my everyday activities: open a jar, slice vegetables, lift a skillet, use the electric can opener (vibrations), wash my hair (raise my arms above my head), blow my hair dry, make my bed, bend over to pull on a pair of pants, pet my cat. Every time I tried, my muscles retracted in pain. I tried to read, but looking down hurt my neck. I tried raising the book up, but it was too heavy for my hands. I tried to sleep, but I couldn't lie on my sides. I tried to lie on my back, but then I couldn't fall asleep. About the only thing I could do was cry. If my bathroom weren't so tiny, I would not have been able to use the toilet. It was excruciating to reach back to wipe. Every second of every day I had to rethink every single thing I did.

If you think my story is awful, I know hundreds of stories that are much worse: stories of mothers who cannot lift their babies, fathers who cannot support their families, and employers who appear at the homes of injured employees, demanding that they return to work. In the midst of unbearable pain, you're thrown into a whirlwind of rules and regulations, forced to deal with insurance companies, doctors, and lawyers, all of whom speak a language you don't understand. I was lucky to have a college education. I had worked for lawyers and have an understanding of the law. Still, the injustice of the system was a shock. I actually faired very well through my ordeal. Many RSI sufferers do not.

My chiropractor couldn't prescribe any pain medication. I could only ease the pain by lying on the floor with my feet in a chair and first applying ice, then, twenty minutes later, switching to heat. I kept calling my attorney, but once I had hired him, I couldn't get him on the phone. I kept leaving messages, begging him to get me some pain medication—to no avail.

My denial waned within weeks. I was running out of money. It was time to tell my family. I knew how difficult it would be for them, living two thousand miles away. Frightful images of what I had become would flood their imaginations. Heck, even I avoided looking at myself in the mirror. My parents were living on a fixed income. They'd carefully managed for a modest retirement. They certainly hadn't factored something like this into the equation. "How long?" They wanted to know. I had no answers to give them. The insurance company had ninety days to review my claim, so I told them three months, hoping that would buy me enough time. I'm so lucky they could help me. I've met others in my situation who have had to live in homeless shelters while trying to recover.

My chiropractor recommended I walk as much as possible to ease the spasms. So, after about a week, I headed down the four blocks to my bank. I barely made it. When a piece of paper slipped from my hands, I had to drop to my knees, then bend to pick it up. A passing woman, aghast at my frailty, stepped around me as if I were broken glass. We are herd animals; we isolate the old and the sick because they attract predators. They endanger the rest of the herd. Still, we hardly ever experience our feral nature. Now, I represented danger, on a very primal level, to everyone who saw me. Others can respond with anger, blame, or downright denial. Still, if you look close, you'll see terror in their eyes.

From then on, I tried to hide my injury as much as possible, which only made it harder on my relationships. RSI is particularly difficult for the people around you. They can see you're in pain, but they can't see why, let alone understand it. Even the disabled community doesn't recognize RSI sufferers as disabled. After all, you're not blind; you can walk. But have you ever tried doing anything without your hands? You use them for everything.

Gavin DeBecker, in his book *The Gift of Fear: Survival Signals That Protect Us from Violence*, writes about why people rubberneck when passing the least little incident in traffic. He says we all want to know how to prevent whatever it is from happening to us—be it a flat tire or a fatal crash.[1] I've found this to be true. It's hard to watch a once vibrant person fall apart. If it can happen to him or her, then it can happen to you. In this light, others' reactions make sense. It took a long time for me to realize it wasn't personal; the people around me just felt helpless.

But I noticed something else too. One day I was in the grocery store, trying to shop. Canned goods were particularly difficult to handle, so I avoided them as much as possible. Still, if I could get them home, they were much easier to deal with once I got into the kitchen. So I stuck to the small cans on the very bottom shelf. I'd lean on the grocery cart, lower myself to my knees, grasp the can with both hands, lean an elbow on the grocery cart, and pull myself to my feet. When I'd gotten to my feet on this particular day, I saw that a woman from across the produce section had been watching me.

Instead of fear in her eyes, I saw recognition. I could tell she didn't know what was wrong with me but understood that whatever it was had changed my life. The compassion in her eyes remains with me to this day. Since I became disabled, I have formed a number of close relationships in a short time with others who have undergone some sort of life-changing event. The experience enriches you in ways that are difficult to accept while you're in the middle of it. But these friends do come, and they stay with you forever.

Ironically, the first MD I saw was the insurance company's doctor. These doctors get the majority of their business from insurance companies, an inherent conflict of interest. Although they are supposed to be objective, they have a clear incentive to minimize the patient's injuries. I did not feel I could get any of my questions answered by that doctor. I sat in a flimsy paper gown while his nurse asked me endless questions about what I did at work, what I did at home, and what injuries I'd had in the past. The whole time I was so nervous, and in so much pain because I was so nervous, that I had to strain to remember anything. The little voice in my head was cursing like a truck driver. Welcome to the whirlwind of the workers' compensation system. This particular doctor was pleasant and thorough and confirmed that I indeed had carpal tunnel syndrome. He recommended treatments and further testing, none of which the insurance company actually allowed me until I took them to court.

Finally, I saw my own orthopedist, who, thankfully, was willing to place a lien on the underlying legal case and see me while I awaited the insurance company's approval of my claim. He was a reassuringly efficient fellow who dictated into his tape recorder like a rapid-fire machine gun while I sat there.

Whatever he paid his transcriptionist, it was not enough. He waived the whole thing off as if he'd seen it before and could take care of everything. More psychology. I ate it up. He suspected I had carpal tunnel syndrome and ordered a nerve-conduction test. He told me to continue seeing the chiropractor but added physical therapy as well.

I'd marked the ninetieth day of the investigation period in red on my calendar. I'm sure it was marked on my parents' calendar as well, as my rent was three times their mortgage payment. When the last day finally came, I assured them I wouldn't need their help any longer. The doctor who evaluated me for the insurance company reported that I was indeed hurt due to a work-related injury. I was a legal secretary with the typing disease. Even to him it was a no-brainer.

On day ninety the insurance companies denied all three claims made against all three employers. They sent me what was clearly a form letter that read,

> Your claim is being denied because
>
> _____.

They left the reason blank! Apparently, this happens all the time.

My attorney's office told me I had to wait until I'd recovered fully before I could go to court to force payment of benefits. By then I realized I had an incredibly complicated disorder. How was I going to survive in the meantime?

It took two lawyers, three hearings, and fourteen months before I finally received any disability benefits. It took another eight doctors, six hearings, and five years to resolve my case. For those first fourteen months, my parents paid my bills. For the remaining four years, I had to live on two-thirds of my usual salary when I had extra medical expenses, endure being followed by a private investigator for the insurance company, and watch many of my relationships crumble under the weight of my RSIs.

Part 1

THE PHYSIOLOGY OF RSIs

Chapter Two

Why It's Important to Educate Yourself about RSIs

There are many reasons to educate yourself about repetitive strain injuries, for recovery as well as prevention. RSIs are complicated, and medical science understands very little about them. Their physiology involves multiple systems, interacting in ways medicine can't entirely explain. Every RSI patient is different, and there are no definitive diagnostics. Treatments are controversial. If you find two doctors who agree on the subject, you're lucky. I didn't. Finding the right practitioner can mean the difference between recovery and a lifetime of disability. What's more, many people don't believe RSIs exist; if you contract one, you will battle at every turn to convince them otherwise: your family, your boss, your doctor, and claims adjuster for the insurance company. Your body and your medical issues will become a legal matter, as most RSIs are contracted at work. Finally, if you contract an RSI, you will be frightened and in pain, and you can't triage yourself while in crisis.

I believe RSIs require a team approach, with the patient playing quarterback and the doctor acting as coach. No one knows where and how you hurt the way you do. Practitioners have all the scientific knowledge, but you are unique—your RSIs are unique. Your personal experience is crucial to successful diagnosis and treatment. This is the most important reason to educate yourself about RSIs.

I am not a doctor. I have no medical or scientific training whatsoever. The physiological descriptions I provide in this book are meant as demonstrations of the complexities of RSIs, not as medical advice or even a presentation of the latest research or the whole picture. I encourage you not only to read these pages and the works cited in the bibliography and on the book's website, but also to conduct your own investigation, talk to your doctor, and question everything.

WHAT IS AN RSI?

Medical science does not know what an RSI is. There is information, but it has yet to be culled, let alone shared, at the practice level. The scientific community has not reached a consensus. Because RSIs seemingly came out of nowhere, there was a long lag time before any research could provide a basis for consensus. The research that exists today remains inconclusive. In the absence of definitive research, clinical data filled the gap, giving rise to syndromes named for their location or for the person who "discovered" them. The result is a hodgepodge of over one hundred different kinds that fall under the heading "repetitive strain injury," or RSI. The most common are carpal tunnel syndrome, cubital tunnel syndrome, radial tunnel syndrome, Guyon's canal syndrome, De Quervain's syndrome, Dupuytren's contracture, focal dystonia, epicondylitis, Raynaud's disease, tendonitis, tenosynovitis, thoracic outlet syndrome, trigger finger, cervical radiculopathy, and reflex sympathetic dysfunction. They are also called musculoskeletal disorders, cumulative traumas, occupational overuse syndromes, repetitive trauma disorders, and a myriad of other things, depending on who's tracking them and why. Sometimes they include back pain; sometimes not. Some back pain is attributable to repeated strain; some is not.

Whether it's called iPod finger, tennis elbow, or text neck, it's the repeated trauma that makes it an RSI. You may not think of the pain in your neck as associated with carpal tunnel syndrome, but many believe the lower cervical spine is the very heart of RSIs. Because of the physiology, once you get an RSI, it can migrate through all of your upper extremities if you're not careful. RSIs are related in the way repetitive motion or static positioning causes them. From my experience, that also indicates how they should be treated as I only truly began to make headway into my pain and functionality once my neck was treated as well. This is particularly problematic when your MD writes a prescription for a physical therapist to treat your wrists, when the problem is in your neck. The physical therapist isn't authorized to work on your neck. RSIs can even cause spinal disc problems. The RSIs in my wrists, elbows, neck, and shoulders were so bad that they pulled on the muscles in my back until they tore a fissure in the very last disc in my lumbar back at the bottom of my spinal column. At least, that's how it was explained to me.

When you have two RSIs at once, which often occurs if symptoms are ignored or improperly treated, it's called a "double crush." I have six: bilateral carpal tunnel syndrome, bilateral radial tunnel syndrome, and bilateral thoracic outlet syndrome.

RSIs are called injuries, but many believe they act more like illnesses because the trauma accumulates over time rather than arising out of one sudden accident, and it can move from the musculoskeletal system into the nerves and other systems of the body. Dr. Peter Mandel of the American Academy of Orthopedic Surgeons says, "These should not be called injuries but ailments."[1] Their symptoms can vary from person to person, occur alone or in combination, and present and disappear or remain constant.

Nowadays, any job requiring heavy use of technology has a manual labor component to it because technological tools have become a large part of workers' everyday duties. These tools include not just computers but also tablets and smart phones. Every business and nearly every job has been affected. The use of technology can also affect us long before we enter the workforce—in school or at play. Becoming educated about RSIs is just plain smart from a preventative standpoint. Among adults in the United States, 75 percent use a computer,[2] 62 percent use a computer at work, 83 percent use a cell phone,[3] and 72 percent text with their phones.[4] The use of e-readers has doubled in less than a year.[5] If you use any of these tools regularly, you're at risk for an RSI.

Parents should also educate themselves about RSIs because US children between the ages of eight and eighteen spend more than six hours a day texting, typing, or playing on some type of computer or electronic device.[6] They are most certainly at risk for an RSI.

Employers should educate themselves about RSIs because the costs are exorbitant. One case can bankrupt a small business. A 2010 National Health Interview Survey found there are approximately 4.8 million people with carpal tunnel syndrome, and 69.4 percent of these cases were attributed to work.[7] The majority of workers who contract RSIs earn more than $50,000 a year,[8] so if you think you don't have to worry because you don't own a poultry-processing plant, guess again. If your employees are using technology, your business is at risk.

Of the workers losing work time due to RSIs, nearly half change jobs within thirty days of diagnosis.[9] RSIs are now the most common cause of physical disability in the world.[10] What would it cost you to lose your best employee or to change jobs? What if you're self-employed or uninsured? Can you really afford not to educate yourself about RSIs?

RSIs are not new. Repetitive motion injuries have been around for a long time. It's who's getting them and how, as well as how many are getting them, that is cause for alarm. Between 1976 and 1983, work-related injuries due to repeated trauma held steady at around twenty-five thousand per year. But since 1987, when PCs became common in the workplace, incidents have risen sharply. By 1994, when the Internet became an essential work tool, repeated traumas had increased by over 1,000 percent.[11] They've been the number one occupational illness in the United States for almost two decades. The Occupational Safety and Health Administration (OSHA) say RSIs have reached epidemic proportions, just as tablets join the workplace, exposing many more to injury. Yet, of all the people I've met over the past dozen years, few are aware that using technology can lead to disability. How can this be?

OSHA has battled to reduce RSIs in the workplace. The media regularly report about carpal tunnel syndrome and BlackBerry thumb. Technology manufacturers include lengthy warnings in their product manuals. The Internet is filled with preventative information. A Google search reveals over 12 million sites discussing carpal tunnel syndrome alone. How can there be such a disconnect between the facts and public perception?

"OSHA is underfunded; they have no way to get the word out about RSIs," says ergonomist Jonathan Bailin. He also cites our reliance on primary care, the general practitioner or family doctor our health-care system sends us to first. They're trained to handle acute illness and test for disease. "They're not very good at chronic illness, and RSI is a chronic condition."[12]

I think there is much more going on here than mere bureaucratic bungling. Beneath the boldfaced statistics, bankrupting medical costs, and large-scale loss of human resources lie very real social and political issues that require a totally new way of thinking. These include a dysfunctional health-care system in which patients no longer trust doctors, a global economy in which our national production capacity is being eclipsed for the first time, and the threat to the corporate bottom line of medically and legally establishing the fact that stress on the job really does cause injury and illness. All of these require a massive retooling of our very notion of how we work. Since most of us RSI suffers cannot write letters, hold the phone, sit through meetings, or march on city hall, we're powerless, and you're left uninformed.

Even when I was working at a law firm, one of the hotspots for RSIs, what I heard about carpal tunnel syndrome in the lunchroom was incredibly dangerous. You get surgery and are back at work in three weeks. In ergonomist Jonathan Bailin's experience, "Surgery is unfortunately not that successful." That nearly half of those who get diagnosed with an RSI change jobs within thirty days suggests that too many patients have gotten surgery, only to find the problem has not gone away, but the insurance coverage has.[13]

The gap starts in the media, which give all the attention to "sexy" syndromes, like BlackBerry thumb and trigger finger. The issue is just too complicated for a thirty-second story in a segment-formatted medium. Plus, a huge media campaign being waged against injured workers goes against the message behind RSIs. Finally, newsrooms are full of people typing on deadlines. I bet a lot of them have wrist and arm pain, and their employers, fearing a costly epidemic in their own organizations, ignorantly try to squelch the stories.

Let's face it: the news isn't what it used to be. Broadcasters were once required to air programming of public interest to maintain their licenses in accordance with the Fairness Doctrine, but that doctrine was repealed in 1987. Budgets have since been slashed, and reporters can no longer afford to do the investigative work for which they were once known. They're now competing not only with cable and Internet outlets but also with entertainment outlets. The press formerly had to corroborate everything it printed using two separate sources. Now entirely unsubstantiated articles appear on the Internet every day. Other outlets then pick those articles up, which means you are relying on an entertainment program to inform you about health issues.

RSIs do get a lot of press, but usually in the form of sound bites that conflict with what the last sound bite said. For years Wikipedia reported, under its "BlackBerry thumb" entry, a study revealing that pain signals could send a "false alarm." Anyone would draw the reasonable conclusion that BlackBerry thumb doesn't cause pain at all—except there's nothing truthful about that conclusion. You'd have to read the fine print about the narrow focus of the study and its complete results in order to understand not to ignore that pain.

PAIN IS THERE FOR A REASON

Ergonomist Bailin finds that patients are resistant. "We're used to thinking the human body is going to heal itself or 'I have to go to the hospital,' but nothing in between. There's a lot in between that still needs to be explained. RSI pain is not going away by itself; it's a warning."[14]

Even if the news accurately and completely reported on RSIs, you'd still ignore the pain anyway. No one wants to stare down the barrel of a serious illness. How long did the health-care industry have to harp about cholesterol before we stopped slathering butter on top of everything we ate? How many people still do? We tend to ignore our pain. Maybe it's our Puritan background; we think our pain makes us weak or that it's not real.

I think we are nation plagued by a "never cry wolf" backlash when it comes to pain. Do you remember saying, "Mommy, I don't feel good. I can't go to school," but she made you go anyway? I found, as an adult, that I had no reference point for accurately measuring my own discomfort. Yet discomfort is how our body tells us something needs our attention. The pain is there for a reason. Don't chase it away or ignore the symptoms.

Perception is vital to the experience of pain. Pain involves complex processes in various centers in the brain. According to David A. Williams, PhD, of the University of Michigan's Chronic Pain and Fatigue Research Center, it includes "your emotional reaction to having something happening in your body."[15] Williams says, "Your conscious awareness of the pain, your memories of previous pain and whether you can handle it or not, all have to come together and be processed in order for you to actually experience pain."[16] That doesn't mean that if you don't process those signals, you're not suffering. You are, and by not being able to perceive this, in the case of an RSI, you're exposing yourself to potentially permanent damage.

We all go to work with a cold or a fever and infect everybody else. So let's redefine acceptable levels of pain right here: if something doesn't "feel good" or "feel right," and you rest or take aspirin and the sensation doesn't go away or it comes back again, that's not normal. Your body requires more rest, or you need to change your diet, or your lifestyle, or your doctor. Or maybe you need to have your head examined (that is also viable). Just don't dismiss the pain. I have met a person who waited twenty years to deal with her RSIs. The longer you ignore your symptoms, the longer it takes to undo the damage. As soon as you begin to notice something amiss, see a doctor. So what if you're wrong and it's nothing? That assumes, of course, that your doctor knows how to treat RSIs.

Despite all evidence to the contrary, many people still do not believe that RSIs exist. This is in part due to scientific studies that are too narrow or whose results are inconclusive. A study at the Mayo Clinic of its own personnel revealed no connection between carpal tunnel syndrome and the computer keyboard. Of course, there are way too many other factors involved to rely on such a study, even if the prestigious Mayo Clinic conducted it. Such factors include whether the subjects had any pain in the first place, whether they had an RSI other than carpal tunnel syndrome, and whether the clinic had ergonomically designed workstations. Dr. Barry Simmons, chief of the Hand and Upper Extremity Service in the Department of Orthopedic Surgery at Boston's Brigham and Women's Hospital, says 90 percent of carpal tunnel cases are "idiopathic,"[17] a word that sounds an awful lot like "made up" to the layperson but that really means "from unknown causes."

The biggest reason to educate yourself about RSIs is that spotting the pain is only the beginning; the challenge comes with trying to do something about it. When the experts don't agree and you are not an expert, navigating this controversial world can be very difficult. You know you're in pain, but the tests, the doctors, the lawyers, the employers, and the insurance company can't find any proof. Your friends and family can see you're hurting, but they don't understand why. My physiological descriptions in these pages are meant as a way to begin to explain what's happening in your body and to communicate that effectively to those around you. When you start to feel that numbness and tingling, what kind of doctor do you see? An orthopedist? A chiropractor? How about a rheumatologist (a doctor who focuses on disorders of the joints, muscles, and ligaments) or physiatrist (a rehabilitation specialist who focuses on how you move, a problem at the heart of RSI)? The news reports don't cover any of that. I didn't even know what a physiatrist was.

Remember that some say RSIs act more like illnesses than injuries. Despite the images presented in carpal tunnel surgery ads, RSIs don't always occur in one place and affect only a bone structure. The surrounding systems can become affected by the original injury, and those effects must be treated as well. RSIs can also injure muscles, nerves, joints, tendons, ligaments, blood vessels, the lymph system, or any combination or even all of them.

Once you injure a muscle through repetitive motion in a cumulative trauma, the surrounding systems can also become traumatized. Undoing the damage can involve a process of relaxing the muscles, which have memory; repairing the nerves and connective tissues, which takes a long time; and unrestricting the blood vessels, where toxins have pooled and aggravated the tissues they feed. This is why surgery is such a controversial treatment for RSIs. Simply widening the carpal tunnel does nothing to heal the muscle, nerve, and tendon if they're damaged as well. It just stops them from being damaged further. Maybe that's why so many people change jobs.

Dr. George J. Piligian, assistant clinical professor of occupational medicine in the Department of Preventive Medicine at Mount Sinai in New York, describes RSIs as a "series of injuries, not localized, but regional, which goes along with the way our bodies are built."[18] Maybe this is why RSIs are so difficult to diagnose. Piligian believes the root of the problem begins with the name given to these conditions: "RSI is a colloquial name. What's repetitive? Which parts of the body? Stress is a little defined term. The only understood part is injury as opposed to illness."[19] Piligian would like to see the classification of these injuries changed. Now each syndrome is identified according to the part affected. So, if your complaints fit the classic definition of, say, tendonitis in the elbow, doctors might not look at your neck. Another reason Piligian gives for the difficulty in diagnosing RSIs is a lack of appropriate physician training, either in medical school or in residency programs, in what constitutes a repetitive strain injury in the first place.

Part of the problem with RSIs is that many patients see the wrong doctor or receive the wrong or ineffectual treatment, and their RSI only gets worse. If you belong to a health-management organization, the referral process alone can cause your RSIs to worsen. Appendix A contains a list of types of practitioners who treat RSIs. Your exact symptoms and what aggravates them should drive which type of professional you see.

BECOME YOUR OWN ADVOCATE

Surgeon and health journalist Atul Gawande advocates a "pit crew" approach to medicine.[20] A pit crew is a team of specialists who work together toward a common goal. They operate from one central location and easily share information. Our current health-care system is so dysfunctional that information does not necessarily travel from one practitioner to another on the same team. That means that sharing this information is part of your job as the quarterback of your health-care team.

I often had to carry one doctor's report to another treating practitioner, hand it to that person, and then ask to discuss it then and there to ensure that he or she read it. Actual communication between my practitioners did not exist at all. I later found other doctors who knew each other and would pick up the phone and chat about me as a patient. But they were young and had gone to medical school together. Thank goodness medical schools are educating their students this way now. Doctors who have been practicing for a while, however, are not used to functioning as a team. It's not their fault; they just weren't trained that way.

When it comes to "soft tissue" injuries, practitioners rely heavily on their patients' reports. If you aren't well versed in the medical descriptions of pain, it's easy for you and your doctor both to become frustrated. Each of the dozen or so doctors I saw asked me to rate my pain on a scale of one to ten. But they never gave me examples of what each number felt like. Pain is so subjective. Some people have a high tolerance for it, whereas others are very sensitive. How a patient is experiencing pain is as important as where. I always rated my pain in the range of five to seven. However, a year or so after I was released from the workers' compensation system, I was visiting a friend in the hospital who had just had back surgery. There on the wall was a pain chart, with little faces under each number and a corresponding expression. I realized from this chart that my pain had in fact been an eight or a nine the entire time.

Soft tissue ailments receive a bad rap due as much to poor communication between practitioners and patients as to deficits in testing and understanding on the medical side. Many patients experience the frustration of having their doctor imply that it's all in their head. Chronic pain patients can easily be labeled chronic complainers, especially when medical science cannot pinpoint what's causing the pain. That's not to say the pain does not exist. It would be more accurate to say that either the test to measure the pain or a full understanding of the pain being experienced does not exist. Sports medicine has actually made the most progress with soft tissue injuries. Professional athletes are usually eager to return to the game, and there's an obvious cost-benefit for them to do so as quickly as possible. If only other employers saw their injured employees as important members of their revenue-generating team, like sports teams do. Of course, athletes are also in top physical condition, and not every employee is.

I define a good doctor as someone who looks at me, touches me, and talks to me like I'm a person. If you think about it, what doctors do—poke, prod, and cut into other human beings—is pretty remarkable. I don't think I would have the stomach for it. It takes a lot of raw nerve to crack open the ribs and touch the heart of another person. I understand that they have to remain objective in order to do their jobs. But I want someone who is more than merely objective; I want a healer. You may prefer someone who is efficient or candid or conservative in his or her approach. In that case, that's the type of doctor you should look for.

You also have to have a certain amount of understanding about your condition before you can select the proper practitioners for you. Some doctors treat RSIs as musculoskeletal disorders, believing they involve only the muscles and joints. Others treat RSIs as neuromuscular problems, believing nerves are the source of the problem. Your RSI can involve either. Mine involved both. When an RSI has become systemic, as mine has, a practitioner who treats the whole body rather than specializes in surgery on a particular body part might be more helpful to you. A rheumatologist specializes in autoimmune diseases. While RSIs are not currently called diseases or believed to be immune responses, some practitioners have had success in looking at them in this way. This is why it's important for you to be educated about RSIs, so that you can communicate, with a level of detail and sophistication, what you're experiencing.

"I hurt" will not help anyone, even though that's all I could say for at least a year and a half. Tracking not only your pain but also your mood, fatigue and activity levels, sleep, and even what you're eating will help. In addition to informing your decision about what type of practitioner to see, this will help you track the efficacy of the treatment you're receiving. Appendix A contains some great resources to help you. Penney Gowan founded the American Chronic Pain Association (ACPA) "to bring everyone together so that they speak the same language, so that they can begin the conversation."[21] Gowan's organization has some terrific communication tools available on its website, including a pain log and abilities chart (www.theacpa.org). A quick glance reveals just how in depth your description should be.

Once you begin tracking your pain and treatment, bring copies of your logs to every practitioner you visit. They will become part of your medical record as well. Make sure you get a copy of every medical report written about you and that every practitioner treating you gets a copy too. Discuss the reports and logs with every practitioner. Get their feedback, even if you already know what they think. It's a good way to make sure that they have read the report. It's also a good way to get your questions answered. Remember, people in health care have very logical minds. When you ask a logical question, it makes sense to them. Responding to their questions with vague, emotional answers doesn't help them do their job at all. If you can't do this by yourself, ask a friend or family member to help you. In the end, these logs and your communications efforts will help medical science learn more about RSIs.

Current thinking in medical science for treating an injury is to fix the underlying mechanical problem or immobilize the specific area to allow it to heal. I saw many practitioners who believed they knew all about RSIs. They could even offer evidence to support their theories. They could have been right, or wrong, or a little of both. The important thing was for me to weigh a practitioner's theory against my own experience. If it fit, I found their treatments helpful. But if it didn't jibe with what I was experiencing, I steered clear. That's not to say that their theories were incorrect. I only offer this as a way of navigating a very complex territory. For instance, my injury was too advanced for immobilization, and lifting weights only aggravated it. With a cumulative trauma, one condition can cause another condition, which can cause a third, which can aggravate the first. How do you fix that? Some people look for a specific place to begin. Since my pain was not localized, I went for treatments that addressed the entire affected region rather than one particular site.

You may wind up seeing a number of specialists for your RSIs, and chances are, they won't agree about causes or treatments. This can actually be a benefit. I leveraged the differing opinions I received to create a system of checks and balances, so that I didn't head too far down the wrong path of any one particular treatment. In my case, many of my treatments lasted twelve months or more. I could ill afford to waste time.

One of the most frustrating aspects of my injury in the early stages—and another reason why educating yourself about RSIs is extremely important—was that I was expected to make important decisions, like whether to have back surgery, without, to my mind, sufficient knowledge, understanding, or mental resources. You can't make judgments about complex medical issues when you're a layperson and have cognitive impairment—which you will if you have chronic pain. By the time you experience RSI pain, you've probably been in pain for much longer than you've perceived.

RSI IS A LEGAL ISSUE

Another reason to educate yourself about RSIs is the workers' compensation system. Although, with all the technology at home as well as at work, it's hard to tell exactly where a person developed an RSI, 67.1 percent of cases are attributed to the workplace.[22] When you get RSIs on the job, they become not just a medical problem but a legal one as well. That these ailments are so difficult to pinpoint and often cannot be proven conclusively only provides ammunition for insurance companies to deny benefits.

Even if your RSI is only partially attributable to work, you're legally obligated to file a workers' compensation claim. If you receive treatment for a work-related injury from your regular health insurance provider, you actually risk committing insurance fraud. Conversely, if your workers' compensation claim is denied because it's not attributed to work, you can then seek care through your health insurance. Once you file a claim, your treatment is prescribed by the workers' compensation system. The workers' compensation insurance company insures your employer. It has a duty to act in good faith to your employer, not you. Under that system, you, as an injured worker, must prove that you are injured and that your job caused that injury. The insurance company can provide whatever treatment it likes, or not, as long as your employer doesn't object. If you object, however, you have to take the insurance company to court to force provision of benefits. That can be a very lengthy and difficult process.

Once in the workers' compensation system, you'll have to discuss RSIs with another group of people who don't understand them: lawyers and administrative law judges. My second attorney was familiar with RSIs because he had once worked for a workers' compensation insurance company. This helped me a great deal. But my first attorney knew absolutely nothing about RSIs, and I needlessly went without any disability benefits for more than a year because of that. When looking for a workers' compensation attorney, find out how many chronic cases candidates have handled. That will give you a good idea of who is capable of handling a complex case. You'll need to run point on your legal case as well. Workers' compensation attorneys don't make a lot of money, so they have to take on a lot of cases in order to turn a profit. It is so easy to slip through the cracks. Make sure you keep copies of every legal document. Keep in regular contact with your lawyer to track deadlines, hearings, and insurance company promises. Follow up on those as well.

There's also a benefit to being able to explain RSIs to your employer. If you work for a small business, even one case of RSI can shut the shop down. Your knowledge of RSIs can benefit your employer tremendously, but take a team approach. RSIs can put an office in upheaval. Work redesign and a preventive approach are far cheaper than an injury, but implementing them means changing minds, and that's not an easy thing to do.

If you develop an RSI, being able to explain your injury to friends and family will help them understand and support you in ways that will help you recover. Catastrophic illness affects everyone around you. It frightens your loved ones and creates tremendous challenges for every relationship. Invisible disabilities are particularly difficult for others to understand. They're also an opportunity to deepen relationships. People often don't know what to say to someone in pain, so they look to the sufferer to lead the way. A thorough understanding of RSIs can help with that.

And if I haven't drawn a serious enough picture, let me tell you where the real devastation of an RSI lies: quality of life. Twelve years later, I still have not recovered 35 percent of my grip strength. No big deal you say? Guess again. It's the little things that give me trouble: opening a jar or a bag of chips, turning a key in a lock, carrying in the mail, washing my hair. I miss certain big things, too, like riding a horse, skiing, running, and taking long trips. I can't have any impact on my back, as in high-impact aerobics, which makes weight control really difficult. Traveling is particularly hard, between carrying luggage and sitting for long periods. Half of my suitcase is filled with stuff to address my RSIs. What if I had small children? I wouldn't be able to pick them up. I can't pet my cat. It hurts when my boyfriend holds my hand.

But the best reason for educating yourself about RSIs is that once you get one, if you don't know what you're dealing with, you're not likely to get help immediately. You won't know what's happening to your body. You will feel betrayed by the very thing you've identified as yourself. You'll dismiss the pain, thinking it will go away. This is the first stage of grief: denial. The truth of the matter is, by the time you feel the pain, you're already well down the road of RSI.

Ergonomist Jonathan Bailin, who is called in at the first sign of trouble to modify someone's workstation, says, "Americans are used to taking a pill; they're not used to having to change their lifestyle in order to improve their health."[23] If you contract cancer, your body shuts down, forcing you to see a doctor, who then gives you a diagnosis. Then you hunker down for the fight. Cancer forces you to face your mortality. There are no such mechanisms with RSIs. By the time your body shuts down, it's too late. As I write this book, I have two close friends with RSIs, both of whom have heard me tell my story over and over again. I have urged both to seek serious interventions before it's too late. Both have taken some steps, but their pain continues. Neither thinks their RSIs will get as bad as mine, even though they both have been experiencing symptoms on and off for years. In the end, your health is first and foremost your responsibility. My RSIs showed me that you can't triage yourself when you're in crisis. You just can't. It's much better to learn what to do in advance—as we do by participating in, for instance, fire drills—so that when a crisis hits, you know what to do and simply respond.

The ACPA's Penney Gowan likens our health to a car: "Its our job to maintain our car, not the dealer's."[24] In the end, educating yourself about RSIs, as well as a preventive-medicine approach to your health in general, is your job, not your doctor's.

Chapter Three

How Can You Become Disabled Just by Sitting at a Computer?

When faced with catastrophic illness, you suddenly have to get up to speed in the middle of your catastrophe. I had to learn a whole new language while lying on the floor with my feet in a chair. To make matters worse, I couldn't hold up a book or look down to read. I'd read a bit, switch positions, read the same passage again, switch positions again, and look up every other word before switching positions again. I had a litany of questions whose answers only confused me more. Finally, I turned to the Internet, where I found more user-friendly explanations. But how do you know what you can trust on the Web?

Sure, there are a lot of dramatic statistics, but they lack citations and credible backup data. Start digging into the research on repetitive strain injuries, and you'll find conflicting or inconclusive results there as well. Patient sites can completely contradict medical ones. RSI product sites are often the worst, providing dramatic statistic about RSIs, in quotes no less, then offering their device as a wonder cure. Some doctors' sites provide answers about surgery when they haven't even examined you. There is no definitive effective treatment. Even the experts don't know. Still, you have to figure out a way to get through this.

There is also an underground subculture of RSI sufferers on the Internet, doing what little they can to form a grassroots movement. They recommend local practitioners and share treatment strategies and work-arounds through a network of local support groups around the world. A list of them can be found under "Support Groups" in appendix A. I found one group that met at a nearby library. I hesitated to go; I thought it would be a whine-and-cry session, and I didn't want any part of that. But I knew I needed to take some control of my life. Knowledge is power, and I had none. Even if they were just a bunch of kooks getting together to share their misery, at least they wouldn't shrink from me. I decided to make the trek.

I walked into that library meeting room to find people moving around like flailing windmills. They paced and stretched, bending their wrists back and forth. They were doing some of the recommended exercises for RSIs that I'd seen on the Internet, but I wasn't prepared for the crazy calisthenics en masse. Everyone in the main library walked by the windows and just stared into the community room at us. We stared back, shouting, "Never hold the phone to your ear with your shoulder!" We must have seemed ridiculous.

When the meeting started, I found this was no whine-and-cry session. In retrospect, the Los Angeles RSI Support Group (LARSI) comprised an extraordinary group of smart, savvy people who were taking matters into their own hands. A computer programmer at NASA's Jet Propulsion Laboratory, who had been stumbling along with his RSIs for a number of years, started the group. The members were well-educated, well-paid professionals. Their ranks included a neuropsychologist from Harvard University, an insurance executive, a city planner, a civil engineer, an operating engineer, two video game developers, a librarian, a systems engineer, and even an actress. Just as RSIs were becoming a political football, these brave pioneers represented a unique and critical component in the discussion of the issue. Nearly everyone had a college degree; most had advanced degrees. Many had been business owners or department managers themselves, so they were sensitive to the employer's side of the equation. A number of them had been earning more than $100,000 a year. They represented a significant loss of human resources.

They met monthly to exchange treatment strategies and information. At each meeting, a health-care practitioner who had successfully treated patients with RSIs came to speak. The speakers understood the level of intelligence in the room, so they presented their own theories about what causes RSIs and why they're so difficult to treat as they would to peers. They brought scientific or clinical evidence to support what they had to say, and we drilled them with questions afterward. In order to speak, they had to have been recommended by a member of the group who had made marked improvement by following their protocols. Yes, they were gaining new patients from the group, but most were excited that someone was interested in what they had to say about their clinical discoveries. We didn't realize it at the time, but we were all at the forefront. I take much of what I write about the physiology of RSIs in this book from those presentations.

Dr. George Piligian is a clinician who has also been working in the trenches, first working with a leader in the field of RSIs, Dr. Emil Pascarelli, at the Miller Institute for Performing Artists, a unique multispecialty clinic designed to diagnose and treat professional musicians and dancers. Piligian expresses a similar excitement when he recalls, "We were pioneering treatment because these disorders didn't have much scientific study devoted to them. Till now there's not been enough research that's been done."[1]

In today's health-care system, it's a rare treat to have a doctor, physical therapist, or yoga instructor spend an hour talking and then answering questions. The discussions were always lively, and strong relationships formed between the practitioners and patients.

The guest speaker at my first meeting was a real eye-opener. Peter Edgelow, a West Coast physical therapist renown for treating thoracic outlet syndrome (TOS), began his speech with a cold slap in the face: "You have to think that what you have is as serious as cancer. While it won't affect the length of your life, it will affect the quality of it."[2]

Little by little, meeting by meeting, I began to get the picture, and it wasn't pretty. Despite my doctors' nonchalance, I discovered I had a terrible, difficult, controversial medical problem. I also came to understand that patients usually get lost in the health-care system while their RSIs grow worse until they become totally disabled. One member of LARSI had been suffering for twenty years: a simple case of De Quervain's syndrome that had been misdiagnosed and then mistreated blossomed into thoracic outlet syndrome and then fibromyalgia, a common end-stage complication of RSI. Fellow sufferers turned out to be my best resource for developing a treatment strategy. I learned that what works for one sufferer does not necessarily work for another. You have to hunt and peck to find the right treatment at the right time for each individual. Understanding how you became injured to begin with is the best place to start.

THE MEDIAN, ULNAR, AND RADIAL NERVES

This and the following chapters present what I learned from those LARSI sessions, which explained RSIs to me in ways that made sense. I provide these explanations not for their medical accuracy but as a way for the layperson to begin to understand RSIs. I believe that my understanding of my condition, as rudimentary as it is, went a long way to allowing me to learn to manage it. At the end of the day, the experts go home with their healthy hands, whereas RSI sufferers do not. We don't get to walk away from the pain, the things we can't do, and the lost quality of life. I found it tremendously helpful to be able to speak about my condition with specificity. Even if my practitioners did not agree with my understanding of my condition, they at least took me seriously. This was true in both the medical and the legal circles. Therefore, I believe it is more important for patients to gain an understanding of the physiology involved than it is for the experts to agree with my explanations.

As I understand it, upper-body RSIs can occur in two general areas: (1) the hands and arms, and (2) the neck and shoulders. These are intimately related regions of the body. An RSI can start in one, for instance, as carpal tunnel syndrome in the wrist, then migrate into the neck, becoming cervical radiculopathy, or vice versa. I'm told that carpal tunnel is the least common RSI. Ground zero for all of them seems to be three nerves—the median, the ulnar, and the radial—all originating in the neck. Those nerves travel from the neck, through the brachial plexus located laterally just inside and under the shoulder, down to the arm, and into your hand. The ulnar nerve runs under your arm, ending in the little and ring fingers; the median nerve runs through the center of your arm, ending in the middle and index fingers; and the radial nerve runs under your upper arm, then along top of your forearm, before ending in the thumb and index finger. For visual thinkers, pictures are provided on this book's companion website (http://www.truthaboutcarpaltunnel.com).

The ulnar nerve is the largest unprotected nerve in the human body, with very little sheathing muscle or bone. That turns out to be a good thing, because injury occurs when the ulnar nerve becomes entrapped. Still, because it is so unprotected, injuries are pretty common. The median nerve is the only one that passes through the carpal tunnel, and because it runs through the center of the arm, it doesn't get injured nearly as often. The radial nerve controls all twelve of the muscles that allow you to extend your arm.

With RSIs, any or all of these nerves can become entrapped in the tight passageways of tunnels and outlets in the brachial plexus, elbow, and wrist. They can also become pinched in any number of places. Or surrounding tissue can swell from overuse and compress nerves, tendons, blood vessels, or other connective tissue. The resulting syndrome is classified according to the location of the compression. Tendons, too, can become trapped, pinched, or inflamed, resulting in tendonitis, tenosynovitis, or tendinosis. What exactly causes RSIs? Dr. Piligian explains: "It's a variety of different pathologies in different tissues. We just don't know."[3] You can see the problems with diagnosis as well as treatment protocols.

Nerves can also become entrapped at the intersection of connective tissues, and even at the conjunction of two muscles, causing intersection syndrome, affecting the thumb side of the forearm. There, two muscles cross over just above your wrist bone. Focal dystonia, the oddest RSI, can occur anywhere in the body and causes involuntary muscle contractions. Musicians often get focal hand dystonia, which causes their fingers either to curl into the palm or to extend outward without control.

Although little is known about the physiological roots of RSIs, the biomechanical ones are very clear. RSIs can be caused by repetitive or forceful movements, sustained or awkward positions, pressure for an extended period (such as resting your arm against the edge of a desk all day), and even vibrations and cold. Have your eyes ever burned from looking at a screen for too long? That's considered an RSI too.

SEVEN TONS OF FORCE

When it comes to the types of movements that correlate to RSIs, both the number of repetitions and the amount of force involved are factors. The number of repetitions can be tracked easily through your device using a stopwatch app and word count. It's the amount of force that's surprising. Industrial engineers lead the research on this, and naturally, no two agree. But Bernard J. Healey, in *Introduction to Occupational Health in Public Health Practice*, calculates the force exerted on a computer keyboard using an average of between three and four ounces per keystroke.[4] Let's apply that to the data-entry worker, who, according to job notice requirements, types forty words per minute, or hits twelve thousand keys per hour. Allowing for breaks, paper shuffling, and other moments when fingers are not flying, let's say the average data-entry worker keys for a total of seven hours a day. That's eighty-four thousand keystrokes, adding up to almost seven tons of force!

The human body simply cannot handle all that repetitive motion. Whether using a keyboard, a mouse, a touch screen, or a joystick, you can overload your muscles and cause serious injury. Be it carpal tunnel from a computer keyboard, tendonitis from a mouse, or cervical radiculopathy from holding the phone to your ear with your shoulder—all are injuries resulting from repeated trauma while using technology.

By far the worst RSI is thoracic outlet syndrome. Nerves, blood vessels, and connective tissues all pass from the arm, through the trunk, and converge in a narrow passageway called the thoracic outlet, located between the base of the neck and the armpit, before entering the spinal column. All this tissue becomes far more compact as it passes through the thoracic outlet. This narrowing wreaks havoc when the tissues going in are already inflamed. The whole arm can become numb, loose circulation entirely, and feel like its on fire all at the same time.

To make matters worse, TOS is the most difficult RSI syndrome to diagnose and treat. Because symptoms are experienced throughout the entire arm, as well as in other places, every TOS sufferer I've met has described a process of eliminating every other RSI before even getting tested for TOS. It is not unusual for that to take a long time. Meanwhile, the disease grows worse and worse as it continues to damage the patient's nerves and circulatory system. I know an RSI sufferer who wound up in a wheel chair because of thoracic outlet syndrome. Bet you didn't think your technology could do that.

Once TOS is diagnosed, treatment can be a marathon up a mudslide. Irreversible impairment from insufficient blood supply in the tissue can occur in twenty minutes. Imagine what happens when your entire arm has been numb for over a year, a common situation in TOS patients. Ischemia can set in, whereby not enough blood flows through the circulatory system, resulting in the buildup of metabolic waste products and the collapse of cell membranes. Worse, when the blood supply is restored, additional damage that's more damaging than the initial ischemia can occur, such as fatal cardiac arrhythmias.[5] No wonder the prescribed surgery—removing the first rib—is so controversial. In this way, the surgery can actually worsen the damage.

Because RSIs accumulate over time, they are sometimes described as occurring in stages. You may have seen the clerk at your local grocer or favorite coffee bar wearing a wrist brace. He or she may have a stage-one RSI, in which the symptom is simply an ache confined to one spot. When symptoms begin to spread and multiply, such as aching and burning in the wrist and forearm, but are relieved by rest, that's described as a stage-two RSI. This is where it gets dangerous, because it is easy to think the symptoms have disappeared. You rest for a few weeks, the pain goes away, and you go back to whatever it was you were doing that caused the injury in the first place. At first, everything seems to be okay. But when the pain returns, that's your body telling you everything is not okay. Those symptoms haven't disappeared; your body is just adapting to them. Be careful they don't find a new place to attack. That's when we get to stage three: multiple symptoms that don't go away, even with rest.[6] When more than one syndrome is involved, it's called a "double crush."

Just as repeating the same movement over time can cause RSIs, holding your body still in one position (called static positioning) can also cause damage. Prolonged standing is a much more obvious cause of pain, but oddly enough, prolonged sitting can be just as dangerous. Nobody believes me when I say I got hurt just by sitting, but it's true. I was at a barbecue one afternoon where everyone else was sitting down to eat except me, because I couldn't. A man offered me a chair, but I had to decline—and then explain. The man said to me, "Lady, I'm a roofer. I have lugged, hammered, and bent over all day long for twenty years and never hurt. You're telling me your back hurts from sitting?" I get this all the time, and the explanation is far too complicated for a conversation at an afternoon party. I didn't just hurt my back; I tore a fissure in the outer covering of one of my discs from sitting too much.

This can happen in all sorts of careers. In fact, long-haul truck driving is one of the top-ten most dangerous professions in part because of the damage to the body caused by prolonged sitting.[7] Turns out, the task of driving puts a tremendous amount of strain on the back. There are accelerations, decelerations, lateral movements, and vibrations running through the body. The constant position changes and instability require the spine to act as a shock absorber. Also, your feet can't provide any stability while you're driving because they're actively engaged manipulating the gas and brake pedals and possibly the clutch. Throw in a stick shift, and you have mayhem. Turns out I should not have been driving at all. Many RSI sufferers lose the ability to drive, which means someone else has to take them to all their doctor appointments, and they see a lot of doctors.

POOR POSTURE IS THE STRONGEST COROLLARY

Admittedly, sitting at a desk doesn't subject your back to the same pressures as driving a truck. At a desk, your own poor posture creates the torque that causes injury. Initially this didn't make any more sense to me than it did to that roofer. Dr. Emil Pascarelli became one of the first to tie posture to biomechanics. Pascarelli worked with musicians and dancers who naturally had a lot of repetitive strain injuries. "Most people wouldn't consider poor posture a serious medical problem, but it can become just that over time," says Pascarelli.[8] He gives a great account of RSIs in his books, but I still had a lot of questions about how posture and biomechanics equaled so much pain for me.

Doctors can describe physiologic processes in the best scientific terms, but I found the most illuminating descriptions came from body workers and massage therapists. It makes sense: as they spend an hour, rather than ten minutes, with their clients, they are used to communicating the complexities of soft tissue to lay clientele. One such person is board-certified massage therapist Lamar Bush. His explanation of RSIs made sense to me immediately. Bush sees that in most RSI cases, posture is generally compromised. He describes how slumped shoulders pull the neck down and forward and the shoulder blades up. This shortens the pectoral muscles and makes it hard for your lungs to take in the oxygen your body needs. The spacious, free-moving cavity of your chest becomes a trap for muscles, connective tissues, nerves, and even blood vessels. Over time, poor posture leads to the "dowager's hump" of the elderly. If you want to know what your own posture looks like, ask a friend to snap a picture of you when you're not thinking about it.

Cardiopulmonary specialist and filmmaker Shelly Atwood takes poor posture one step further, describing how it constricts your diaphragm as well, forcing you to breathe into your chest, filling only 25 percent of your lungs' capacity. Over time, this affects the sympathetic (fight or flight) and the parasympathetic (rest and relax) nervous systems. Atwood explains how she likens these two systems working as a dial, "not two separate dials, but one, where they balance each other out."[9] Atwood says that when we breathe with our diaphragm, we stimulate our vagus nerve, which taps into the parasympathetic system and calms us down. The vagus nerve is the longest of the cranial nerves and has the widest distribution in the body. Many consider it the master nerve. It runs from your brain, along your spine, under the lungs, and down into your stomach.

Chest breathing, on the other hand, says Atwood, revs your fight-or-flight mechanism too high. It increases cortisol and carbon dioxide levels, while decreasing oxygen levels. Eventually, your body becomes more acidic. That sets up a situation where things become more inflamed in the body. In her upcoming documentary series *Breathe*, Atwood says that the vast majority of adults are chest breathers. She describes how to teach yourself to breathe with your diaphragm: put one hand on your chest, the other on your belly and breathe. When your diaphragm is working, it pushes the belly in and out. "It's about practicing," says Atwood. "It's not like you can just become aware of it, and expect it to be that way. You have to practice, just like with your posture."[10]

As anyone who's ever tried to change his or her posture knows, it's not that simple. Ann Cuddy illuminates the interconnection between posture, body language, and our sense of ourselves in her TED talk.[11] Mere "practice" cannot correct the myriad of psychosocial components of posture. Picture yourself sitting in front of your computer. If you're hunched over the keyboard, peering at the screen, or lying back in your chair with your feet stretched out, you're in poor posture. What about the teenager slouched on the sofa engrossed in his video game? Or the frustrated mother at the supermarket texting her children while trying to push the cart? These are all very emotional positions, filled with body language. They indicate a high level of engagement, the new marketing holy grail. They're the responses these tools were designed to elicit.

Holding the phone to your ear with your shoulder does the same thing to your posture that slouching does; it just torques your body to the left or to the right, instead of forward. Hold your phone to your ear with your shoulder in front of a mirror, and you'll see just how much you're collapsing your chest and pulling on your postural muscles. Now imagine what that does to your lungs, blood vessels, and nerves. Cell phones have made this problem so much worse because they are thinner than the old phones.

Most researchers agree that overworking one part of your body while holding another part in one position wreaks twice as much havoc on soft tissues as either activity by itself. When you slump over for a long period, the body's amazing adaptability comes back to haunt you. I did not know this, but your muscles actually hold your skeleton up, not the other way around. Your musculature acts like an intricate pulley system. Its tension holds your bones together. But the tension has to be correct. Muscles can contract by themselves, but they can't lengthen by themselves; they rely on another muscle or set of muscles to act in opposition to the first muscle in a process called reciprocal inhibition. One muscle, called the agonist, engages, pulls on, and stretches another muscle, called the antagonist. Massage therapist Bush says, "When one muscle is angry at one end, the other muscle becomes angry at the other end as well."[12] The correct tension is lost, and instead of holding up the skeleton, the musculature starts to pull on it in all sorts of damaging ways.

When a muscle is allowed to work and rest, work and rest, the range of motion of that muscle group is maximized. This is why exercise is so good for you. But when a particular muscle is not allowed to go through that process, to relax after it contracts, it begins to shorten on one end, and its range of motion becomes compromised. Slumping over a computer or a cell phone or leaning eagerly forward while playing a video game for hours on end prevents your chest muscles from resting or relaxing. They become shortened near the ribs. Slowly, over time, they can't quite reach up to your neck as they were designed to do, so the neck is pulled down and forward. The shoulders fall along with it. This is why my shoulder froze.

FROZEN SHOULDER

Bodyworker Lamar Bush described the shoulder to me as a joint consisting of three bones, nine muscles, and five tendons. That's why it has such a wide range of motion. A shoulder becomes "frozen" when one or more of the tendons, usually the subscapularis, become damaged. The subscapularis, a pivotal tendon, sits underneath the shoulder joint. From the pictures, it looks like the shoulder merely rests on it. Apparently, there's much more to it than that. Bush explains, "The subscapularis tells the other muscles in the shoulder girdle, 'Hey, I can't work. I'm under repair. Everyone else stop working,' and the whole shoulder locks up." When one muscle stops working, it signals the other muscles to stop working too. "Everybody tries to repair at the same time," says Bush, "but the situation is not repaired; it gets worse"—because muscle, bone, and tendon are not the only things involved in RSI. [13]

Another resource that helped my understanding of RSIs and the complex inner workings between muscles, connective tissues, and nerves is the elegant explanation contained in Deane Juhan's *Job's Body*. Also a massage therapist, Juhan writes, "Connective tissue called fascia wraps around muscles, bones, internal organs, nerves, and blood vessels. In fact, connective tissue envelops literally every cell in your body."[14] Fascia is fibrous; it forms in layers, binding some structures together and allowing others to slide smoothly over each other. Made of collagen fibers that form a wavy pattern, fascia is quite flexible and able to move in multiple directions.

The amazing thing about connective tissue is that it's all made from the same basic substance. Whether it's hard bone or the viscous synovial fluid surrounding your nerves, the difference lies in the crystallinity of its molecular structure rather than its chemical content. It acts like a living ocean, flowing throughout your entire body, morphing from sheets into chords into layers into complex webbings, writes Juhan. [15] "The entire connective system is large enough, complex enough, sophisticated enough, and important enough to our survival to be regarded as one of the vital organs of the body." [16]

Although made of the same basic substance, each type of tissue works in a completely different way. Fascia can be held together by fat cells, under one mechanism, or synovial fluid under a completely different mechanism. Bush likens it to oil in a crankcase: "This ground substance can lock up between layers. It can get dehydrated and set up like cement." [17] When these tissues do slide against each other, as they must in order for you to move, they form adhesions. Your every movement then damages your tissue. Here's where the vicious circle begins: every time you move, you create scars and pain. So you stop moving, making your connective tissue more rigid. With loss of motion comes less heat, as movement generates heat in the muscles. With less heat comes more loss of motion because cold muscles don't move as freely as warm ones. But that's not all.

Muscles also act much like the heart, pumping blood, while the rhythmic tensions and contractions of the muscles massage the internal organs. Under normal conditions, when your muscles stretch and contract, they help blood move through your veins and arteries. But when a muscle is overworked, it doesn't stretch. Then the muscles around that first muscle also stop stretching; soon the entire area is not getting enough circulation. This is where the numbness comes from. You're cutting off the supply of not only oxygen but nutrients and hormones to the whole area. And just as blood vessels bring food to cells, they take away cellular waste. Chronically overworked muscles produce far more toxins. With the surrounding blood vessels also constricted, they can't remove that excess waste. Juhan draws a very dire picture: "The excess toxins gather in pools, making it even harder for blood, nutrients, and hormones to reach the underfed muscles." [18]

Growth hormones can regenerate damaged muscles, but, as just discussed, those hormones can't reach the tissues that need them because the blood vessels are constricted. "A cuff effect steps in to stop circulation in the limb entirely, and the muscle becomes so weak it can't work at all until enough blood returns to nourish it," adds Juhan. [19] This is what happens with thoracic outlet syndrome and what makes it so severe. How can you relax a muscle that can't work? Where does all this contracting stop? Unfortunately, we haven't even begun to describe all the damage that's occurring.

Muscles are also sensory organs. They provide data to your brain via the nerves. The same oxygen shortage and waste buildup that together damage the muscles also damage the nerves. This is where the numbness and tingling comes from. The constantly contracted muscles surrounding a nerve entrap it in swollen, frozen muscle. This puts pressure on the nerve, and when you get to nerve damage, you've got a whole other ball of wax. When chronically pressured, a nerve finds it harder to send and receive signals. Here, Juhan gives us some data so that we can put this into perspective: "Some researchers estimate that five pounds of pressure for five minutes on a nerve trunk [main stem of a nerve] can reduce its transmission efficiency by as much as 40 percent."[20] Remember that earlier force calculation I gave you? At forty words per minute, the nerve trunks in your fingers receive sixty-seven pounds of pressure per minute! Cumulative pressure can be just as bad as sustained pressure if the muscles never relax in between. Under those conditions, it's a wonder your brain receives any signals from your muscles at all.

For those of you who like to text, here are some sobering statistics: According to the Pew Research Center, the average American teen between the ages of twelve and seventeen sends sixty text messages a day.[21] Nielsen says it's more like one hundred.[22] At 160 characters per text, with three ounces of force per character, that's thirty pounds of force per text! As a parent, do you know how many texts your teenager sends a day? If it's sixty, that's just under one ton of force your child is exerting on her fingers per day.[23] And that's just texting. American kids between eight and eighteen now spend around seven hours a day consuming media on technology devices—"almost the amount of time most adults spend at work each day, except that young people use media seven days a week instead of five," says the Kaiser Family Foundation.[24] This means that every time they watch a video, play a game, use the computer for homework, watch TV, or play music, they're pressing those keys at three ounces of force every time.[25] When they're not pressing keys, they're hovering their thumbs over the keypad, which is much worse, their heads hanging down, pulling on their neck. How can your soft tissue not be inflamed?

Once entrapped, the motor nerves start sending garbled signals to the brain. This accounts for my mysterious typing errors. Worse, they can stop sending any signals at all. To survive, muscles actually require electrical energy (signals) from their motor nerves every bit as much as they require oxygen and blood. When they stop receiving signals from their motor nerves, muscle cells waste away. After three to four months, a muscle can return to normal function once the signal resumes. But after four months, the muscles are only partially recoverable. Here's Juhan again with some more sobering data: "After 1 1/2 to 2 years, the cells break down altogether and are replaced by fatty connective tissue, and nothing can regenerate them."[26] It was easily two and a half years before my trapezius muscle began to relax. It was seven years before I could really say that pain wasn't central to my every thought. This is why time is critical in RSIs. The longer it takes to diagnose and find effective treatment, the greater the chance your muscles and nerves will become permanently damaged.

Meanwhile, your hands are still pounding those keys because you're in denial that anything is wrong and because our entire world runs on technology.

The way I learned to type in the first place was wrong—all wrong. I was taught the QWERTY keyboard method, originally designed for use on manual typewriters. The keys on manual typewriters were heavy and took far more force to press. But you also stopped at the end of every line you typed to reach up and manually return the carriage to its leftmost position. This created a very small, very frequent, very necessary break. Although computer keyboards require much less force, they don't have that break built in. They became a biomechanical disaster. Furthermore, my typing teacher told us to hover our fingers over the keys and never let them venture far from the "home row." On a typewriter, that meant you could easily rest your fingertips on the keys themselves as they were much less sensitive than computer keyboards and could support the weight. But you can't do that on a computer keyboard and certainly not on a touch screen device. Watch people reading e-mails or text messages off a phone; their hands are poised over the device while they read. That requires them to hold their fingers, hands, and forearms up ever so slightly, but hold them up just the same. That's static positioning, and it's working their muscles into exhaustion. If you think that's surprising, consider piano players—their technique hasn't changed since Beethoven. I've met two people who retrain typists to work more efficiently with less injury; both are concert pianists who were forced to learn a new technique themselves.

RSIs have ended promising careers, whether in the concert hall or on the rock stage. If your child is texting sixty times a day and practicing the drums for another two hours a day, you can see how a disaster is in the making.

This slow creep and intricate physiology is why RSIs are so hard to cure. You have to learn first what you're doing that's hurting your body and then learn every way that you're doing it. One of those former concert pianists came to the LARSI group from Australia and offered to give us a free demonstration of his new technique. During his presentation he asked us all to stand and raise our right arms. I'll never forget the look on his face; he was speechless. We were all using the entire right side of our bodies to simply lift our arms. That's how bad our RSIs had become—literally everything we did exacerbated our injuries. This is why finding a suitable health-care practitioner as soon as possible is so crucial to recovery.

Chapter Four

When You Don't Get Proper Treatment, Your RSI Gets Worse

My chiropractor had showed me how to get out of bed by rolling over onto my side and pushing myself up with my hand. At first, the pain in my back, neck, and shoulders was so intense I didn't even feel the pain in my hands. Then one morning, when I pushed down on my mattress to sit up, my wrist gave way. How was I to get up? I was losing body parts by the day. I had stopped working, but my repetitive strain injuries were getting worse! One afternoon at a taco parlor, when I picked up my soda it slipped through my hands and fell to the floor! That terrified me.

Because I waited until my shoulders had frozen before I stopped working on a computer, sitting and typing was no longer the problem. Whereas typing was the original cause, I learned, now the effects were the problem. I was told RSIs act more like illnesses than injuries in that they spread. Just as one damaged muscle tells the other muscles around it to stop working through reciprocal inhibition, damaged muscles in turn tell surrounding nerves that they're not working correctly either. Those nerves tell the surrounding blood vessels, the blood vessels tell the hormones, and so on. Every system in your body checks itself for performance and then communicates that information back into the system in what I'll call a feedback loop.

A second feedback loop involves the muscles, nerves, and brain. Every time you move a muscle, the nerves send signals from the brain down to the muscle: Hey, how'd you do? Then the muscle sends a signal back up the nerves to the brain. When damaged by repetitive microtraumas, the muscle will tell the brain that it didn't perform the task very well. What does your brain do? It tells the muscle to work harder next time, making your muscles contract even more. I'm sure it's more complicated than this, but you see how the effects of RSIs become the problem. Surrounding muscles are asked

35

to help the damaged muscle out, increasing the extent of the injury. Nerves are told to talk more loudly to the muscle in the event of signal loss, overexciting your neurological system. This is why we were all using the entire right side of our bodies to lift our arms. This is also where a third feedback loop gets involved.

CHEMICAL IMBALANCES AND CHRONIC PAIN

Once the insurance company denied my claims, my attorney told me I had to wait until my condition improved before he could go to court to enforce my benefits. This was not true. Apparently lawyers prefer to handle workers' compensation cases this way so that they only have to argue all the issues once. But an injured worker can set a hearing to determine benefits at any time following the ninety days of determination after filing a claim. Since the workers' compensation system controls by law how much attorneys can charge an injured worker, theirs is a volume business, and the quality of representation suffers. Most cases are pretty simple, and so an attorney can practice workers' compensation law for years without sufficient knowledge to prosecute a more complex case. RSI cases require a much greater level of sophistication, legally as well as medically. At the time I was in the system, it wasn't that unusual for a workers' compensation attorney not to be familiar with RSI cases. Now, it seems, nearly everyone in the system has run across multitudes of them.

Even though the insurance company denied my claim, it still scheduled a deposition for me at its attorney's offices. I hadn't been in a law office since I stopped working and so was wholly unprepared for what happened next. As soon as I heard the ping of the elevator doors opening, a flood of memories overwhelmed me. My throat swelled up. I couldn't breathe. I got dizzy as I stepped into the lobby and leaned against a wall for support. There I faced rows and rows of secretarial desks, all stacked high with files and tapes to be transcribed. I went into a full-blown panic attack. Needless to say, this panic sent massive signals throughout my neurological system, which in turn tightened every muscle in my body, increasing my pain levels.

The insurance company scheduled the deposition hoping to prove I wasn't in any pain at all. Instead, I gave my answers while lying on the floor with my feet in a chair. I couldn't answer the questions. I couldn't think. In less than an hour, the insurance company's attorney halted the proceedings and actually suggested to my attorney that I file a psychiatric claim. In the workers' compensation system, psychiatric claims are a separate injury, which for me meant another ninety days of investigation and another three months without disability benefits. At the previous Los Angeles RSI Support Group meeting, the guest speaker had been an attorney experienced with handling RSI cases and achieving the best patient outcomes. He told me the insurance company could be taken to court at any time to enforce disability benefits and a myriad of other things, including treatment, which is often a legal issue in RSI cases within the workers' compensation system. I fired my attorney after the deposition.

I hired the attorney who spoke at the Los Angeles RSI Support Group. He immediately set a hearing regarding my disability benefits, though the court was so backed up it took three months to get a hearing date. When my lawyer found me on the day of the hearing, I was having another terrible panic attack. It's a good thing workers aren't actually allowed in the hearing rooms. My attorney told me the insurance company hadn't even opened my file. It didn't even bother to raise a defense; it just refused to pay. The California workers' compensation system was so backed up that insurance companies were denying as much as they could and waiting for workers to litigate, betting that they wouldn't. My research shows that this is still the case in California and in most states in the union. My attorney, in fact, never argued anything in front of a judge. He merely met with the insurance company's lawyers; they all went off into a room and worked it out. The insurance company agreed to pay me in full, then didn't send the check. We had to take the company to court a second and third time before it did pay me. The whole process took fourteen months.

You would think that my anxiety would abate after I began receiving disability benefits, but once you have one panic attack, it seems your body becomes conditioned to them so that every time you feel under threat, you have another one. From my experience battling anxiety, I learned there are different forms: generalized anxiety, where you just worry all the time; anticipatory anxiety, where you worry about worrying; and panic, where you've worried so much that your physiology actually becomes convinced you're going to die. All of these chemically aggravate RSIs. I was eventually diagnosed with severe depression and severe anxiety as a result of my injuries.

Here's the fight-or-flight response again. It kicks in whenever the brain receives a signal similar to one that occurred during a frightening episode in the past. The more frightened we were, the more easily those signals trigger us, and the more anxious we become. The fight-or-flight response also kicks in when you're experiencing pain. Pain puts the fight-or-flight system into a state of red alert for the duration of the pain. Adrenaline gets released, sending more blood to the muscles. The problem is that, as pain is an internal stressor, there is nowhere for you to run. The adrenaline doesn't get burned up; in fact, it sensitizes the body and brain so that the next time the fight-or-flight system gets triggered, even more adrenaline is required to produce what the brain perceives to be the desired effect.[1] Cortisol also gets released, which increases the body's sensitivity to adrenaline and can aggravate the fight-or-flight response.[2] You wind up in a constant state of vigilance and anxiety, which naturally aggravates all those chronically contracted muscles. Even worse, the release of these neurotransmitters actually inhibits the immune response, slowing healing down.

What if the pain is constant? Lasting years? Then what happens? Overloaded with adrenaline, the flight mechanism is never able to step in and calm you down. If you're a chest breather, the vagus nerve isn't getting triggered to step in either. The constant pain is still triggering adrenaline. The two systems bounce you up and down, searching for a homeostasis that won't interfere with your natural healing process. When these hormones are in your bloodstream for an extended period, the body stops digesting food and starts digesting cells. How's that for a loop?

Pain triggers an adrenaline and cortisol rush, which in turn triggers muscle tension. Chronically tense muscles, in turn, make too much lactic acid, and the chronically constricted blood vessels can't carry the excess away. "When sodium lactate [lactic acid] gets into certain areas of the brain, it induces panic attacks in patients predisposed to anxiety."[3] Anxiety, in turn, increases muscle tension, producing more lactic acid and more panic attacks. Cortisol is the natural version of steroids, and as anyone who follows sports knows, they rev you up. When cortisol is going all the time, adrenal fatigue sets in. That's how RSIs affect your hormones.

CHRONIC PAIN IS NOT JUST ACUTE PAIN
THAT LASTS A LONG TIME

Let's return to Dr. David A. Williams of the Chronic Pain and Fatigue Research Center at the University of Michigan. Trained as a clinical psychologist, he's been studying chronic pain for thirty years. "Chronic pain is a different animal. There's a lot of changes that occur in the body as it transitions from acute pain to a state of chronicity," he says.[4] We are just now learning about some of those changes in the field of pain research.

There are three classes of chronic pain: musculoskeletal (e.g., the pain associated with a broken arm), neuropathic (e.g., the nerve pain associated with diabetic neuropathy), and centralized pain (e.g., the diffused pain associated with fibromyalgia). Musculoskeletal pain is largely in the periphery of the body—at the end of the line, as it where. It's usually revealed by X-rays or MRI scans, and the evidence is pretty easy to find. Neuropathic pain is in the nerves themselves. It's harder to find because we don't have as many tools for seeing damaged nerves as we do for looking at muscles and bones. Still, some forms of neuropathic pain are generated from a specific location, and so we can use other tools to draw enough conclusions to provide effective treatment. The third type, centralized pain, has eluded science until recently. Centralized pain occurs largely in the central nervous system. Currently there are fewer ways to identify centralized pain, and agreement does not exist as to the best methods to diagnose its presence.

Medications, treatments, and interventions that work for one type of pain don't work for the others. Williams emphasizes, "There are interventions for all three, you've just got to match your pain to the right intervention."[5] This means that if you've been given something to treat your pain and its not working, rather than ask for a higher dosage, discuss with your doctor whether it might be the wrong type of treatment. Opiates don't always work; neither do nonsteroidal anti-inflammatory drugs. This is where being able to describe your pain in detail helps.

"The central pain concept has begun to be studied more in the last five years," says Williams. "It's a newer concept." Williams explains what makes centralized pain more difficult to track: "All pain has both a peripheral nerve and central nerve component to it. But with centralized pain, it's real hard to find any injury in the periphery."[6] This explains a lot about fibromyalgia, which can be an end-stage complication of RSI. This also explains all that mysterious pain patients feel that doctors can't locate.

COMPLICATIONS OF IMPROPER OR UNTIMELY TREATMENT OF RSIS

An end-stage complication is the result of one injury or disease's causing a second injury or disease that's equally debilitating as the first one, if not more so. RSIs can lead to a number of these complications, including fibromyalgia, reflex sympathetic dystrophy, chronic fatigue, sleep disorders, and drug addiction. Williams understands why fibromyalgia has been so controversial: "Most of the medical profession has been geared toward finding things they can see, finding the pathology in the periphery. With central pain conditions, we're finding that's only part of the story. When alterations in the central nervous system help to maintain the pain, there may be no easy way to get out of it."[7]

This view represents a paradigm shift in chronic pain management. It explains something RSI patients notice right away: two different people can have the same syndrome but not have the same pain. One has more centralized pain, the other more musculoskeletal pain. Those patients need different treatments. When there is an injury and centralized pain, Dr. Williams emphasizes, "that patient needs treatment for the injury *and* for the centralized pain."[8] For patients who have been told it's all in their heads because their doctors can't find a source for their pain, this research is a tremendous relief. Here, Dr. Williams becomes emphatic: "A mistake medical doctors often make is to assume that if pain does not resolve then it must be related to a psychiatric condition."[9] In fact, it may be due to a mismatch between the type of pain and the treatment. Williams, who has seen patients in chronic pain clinics forty hours a week for twenty years, points out, "There is strong evidence that the multidisciplinary approach is superior for the management of chronic pain. Good pain care involves a cooperative team of people with differing expertise."

On the other hand, Williams also sympathizes with the difficulties doctors encounter with patients. "A patient may hold a strong belief about what they think they need (e.g., that an opiate is the best thing for pain). If someone, say with centralized pain, thinks that an opiate is the only thing that will work, frustration and conflict can arise between the patient and the provider." He points out that education, a rational diagnostic and treatment process, and a shared (i.e., doctor-patient) treatment plan can help reduce the patient's anxiety and improve long-term pain management. But, Williams adds, "bio-chemically anxiety is very different than fear. Anxiety can also be telling you you're not doing it right yet, that you may need to make some additional behavioral changes."[10] Clearly, pain management requires a cooperative approach. Reliance on drugs alone is not an effective solution.

Fatigue, physical and mental, becomes a huge factor with chronic pain. The physical fatigue makes sense: because you can't do as much when you're in pain, you become deconditioned, which leads to further physical fatigue. But processing pain takes up a lot of resources in the brain. If you're trying to keep up your daily routine and processing pain at the same time, you're going to lose brainpower. This cognitive impairment is an important aspect of pain that you should be relaying to your doctor.

In addition to fatigue, I developed another end-stage complication: a sleep disorder. Excessive cortisol and adrenaline can cause sleep disturbances. I had always slept on my sides, but once I was injured, my shoulders hurt too much to bear any weight. Yet I could not fall asleep on my back. I didn't sleep at all until I was given psychotropic medication after the first nine months. From there, I developed a nagging sleep disorder that stayed with me long after my musculoskeletal pain had become manageable. My problem with sleep was cyclical. In the first stage, I could not fall asleep for several hours. In the second stage, I fell asleep, only to wake up in the middle of the night for several hours. In the third stage, I would sleep ten hours a day. And then the cycles would start all over again. In physical therapy, I met a woman who had been run over by a truck. The only position she could tolerate for even a few hours at a time was standing up. She slept leaning into a corner in her dining room.

Another common end-stage complication of chronic pain is drug addiction. When doctors cannot stop the pain or fix the peripheral injury, the last resort is to implant a morphine pump in your body. That, to me, says you are so far gone, they don't even want to spend the money on nurses and therapy for you anymore. There's nothing more to do but wait for you to die. Suicide is another end-stage complication of RSI. Some studies have shown chronic pain patients to have twice the incidence of suicide.[11]

The drug addiction less talked about in connection with chronic pain is that which occurs after prolonged use of psychotropics. Antidepressants and anxiolytics are meant to be taken for the short term. But when your RSI becomes chronic and your workers' compensation case drags on for years, the psychosocial pressures become extraordinary, and without relief of the external factors, psychiatrists can only manage your symptoms, which naturally get worse over time. Among the medications prescribed to me for anxiety were clonazepam, olanzapine, and quetiapine, in succession, not together. These are all drugs made for much more serious mental illnesses, and although they were prescribed in very low doses, they are extremely potent. Each worked for a time, and then the anxiety would come back even more furiously than before. I admit that it was partially my fault: I didn't want to take the drugs and would stop once I got my anxiety under control. I probably made it worse, but the side effects scared me. I developed prolonged dry mouth, which leads to bone loss and had to be treated by a dentist, along with a myriad of other conditions. It took me nearly a year to wean myself off of quetiapine with the help of a professional. Each time I tried taking a lower dosage, I experienced what they call a "bounce": the effects mitigated by the drug, in this case anxiety and sleeplessness, would get worse.

The other complication I feel compelled to talk about isn't end-stage at all. It's called secondary gain, and it's where a patient derives some benefit from his or her injury, such as being relieved from a job with a bullying boss. The workers' compensation system is largely built on this idea of secondary gain. So are employer's reactions to workers' RSI complaints. It's a tough issue to talk about because it is there; it's just not the only thing there. It's hard to self-access secondary gain. I did find my job soul crushing. I didn't like all the lying and injustice that goes on in our legal system or the fact that many of the lawyers I worked for benefitted from others' pain. Still, I did not want to endure unimaginable pain simply to get out of a job. I would have preferred to find another source of income. And I lost so much money in the process.

If you're the major caregiver for a loved one who has RSIs and you think you observe some secondary gain, approach with caution. You could be wrong. Your loved one could feel you're not giving him or her the needed support. But also watch for enabling. I strongly believe that the key to recovery from RSIs is finding that sweet spot where the patient is able to do something without overtaxing him- or herself. That is very difficult to do; with RSI, functionality is a moving target that changes daily. One day you may be able to read a book without much pain at all, but the very next day, you may not be able even to lift the very same book. If you're doing everything for your RSIer, you might want to reconsider that tactic.

It's hard to feel hopeful when you don't ever get to see yourself do something you did before you became injured. By taking over everything from your RSI sufferer, you're also robbing him or her of that very important experience. It's vital not only mentally but also physically. This is where muscle memory will save the sufferer. I strongly believe that finding the things I could still do is part of what helped me learn to manage my RSIs. It allowed me to see the parts of me that had not died. It gave me hope, encouraged me to go on, and gave me a foundation upon which to rebuild my life.

Chapter Five

Ergonomics Alone Cannot Prevent RSIs

You probably think you're familiar with ergonomics. It's become a household word. You may even have had an ergonomist come into your workplace and give you a new keyboard or, if you're lucky, a new chair, when what you really need is a new desk, but your employer doesn't want to spend all that money; besides, your desk matches every other desk in the office, and it looks nicer that way. I've heard many such complaints from repetitive strain injury sufferers, but let's focus on you, your job, and your health. Chapter 10 focuses on employers.

Ergonomics, strictly interpreted, is the science of work. It studies how the tool fits the user, how the user uses the tool, how the worker fits the job, and how the specific tasks of a job are arranged. It includes the fields of psychology, engineering, biomechanics, industrial and graphic design, and even something called anthropometry, or the measurement of human individuals. According to the International Ergonomics Association, there are also cognitive ergonomics, organizational ergonomics, and environmental ergonomics.[1] I include this list here because all of these considerations are important in evaluating how well you're doing you're job and how well your job can be performed by any human.

An ergonomist is called to your workplace for two reasons: something about the work your employer has you doing is causing you pain, and something about the way you're doing that work is causing you pain. Both have to be fixed in order for your pain to stop. That requires partnership. Chapter 10 discusses the first problem. The second problem really comes down to whether the tools and the job fit you and how you are performing the tasks.

In terms of how the tool fits the user, well, nearly everything can be considered a tool. For a long time everything, from staplers to airline seats, was made to fit the scientifically median human body: a 5′2″ man. This means that nothing fit anyone very well, and as anyone who's ever bought a pair of jeans knows, it's all about the fit. In a way, the rise of RSIs helped change all that as industrial design has worked to ensure comfort and safety in the workplace in the name of productivity and profit. So now, for under $100 you can get an ergonomically correct office chair, meaning one whose height, seat angle, back support, and—the one everyone forgets—armrests are adjustable. It's better to have no armrests than for them to be too high. In the latter case, you either have to raise your shoulders or squeeze your arms close to your body, which just makes everything worse.

When selecting ergonomic products remember, it's about fitting the tool to the user, not what your neighbor says. You may have to try a lot of products before you find the right one for you. Look for as many adjustments as possible. Still, just buying the right chair, or wrist rest, or telephone headset won't protect you from getting hurt.

When your productivity begins to wane because there's a weird ache in your hand or arm or elbow, the ergonomist your employer calls in should evaluate not only your workstation but also your posture and keyboarding style, in addition to a host of other things that reveal how you use your various tools to perform your job. Greg Dempster is one such ergonomist, and his story provides a very clear illustration of what using a tool correctly means.

GREG'S STORY

I first met Greg at the Los Angeles RSI Support Group (LARSI). He had been training as a concert pianist since he was a child. When he was eighteen, he was preparing to audition for conservatory when he got badly injured. He had been practicing a technically difficult passage of Chopin's Ballade No. 1 in G minor when there was a pop in his right wrist. It was so loud his mother heard it in the next room. "All of a sudden, my thumb wouldn't move. It didn't hurt, but I couldn't move my thumb anymore,"[2] says Greg. It was the late 1970s, and RSIs didn't exist yet. Over time, he developed bursitis in both shoulders and "tore something" in his left hand. Off and on, for a few years, he would reinjure his left hand, rest it until the pain went away, and go back to playing. Greg tells a by-now familiar story: "I didn't even know I was injured. My first teacher pretended she didn't know what was going on. I tried to pretend there weren't any aches and pains."[3] RSIs have been a dirty little secret in the highly competitive world of classical music for a very long time.

Not until Greg began studying in college did he confront his injury. His teacher was a leading expert nationally on musician injuries in the 1980s. She could tell just from Greg's posture and technique that he was injured. She told him she could not only help him get rid of his pain but also increase his technical ability. She sent Greg to a master class at a piano institute that specialized in retraining pianists. "The thing that convinced me to commit to this retraining was that every night one of the faculty members would give a recital. It was at those recitals that I heard the most astounding, brilliant, stunning players I've ever heard in my life."[4]

Students have been trained to play the piano using a style developed in the academic conservatory system in the mid-nineteenth century. Most pianists can trace their method all the way back to Beethoven. Turns out, the piano technique of Beethoven's time violates every biomechanical aspect there is.

In his first six weeks working with this new teacher, Greg's injuries went away. His retraining took a long time it was years before he understood the technical approach. "But once I did," Greg raves, "I gained control over the expression of my playing that absolutely nothing else can give you. The piano finally became a voice for me."[5] Greg has been injury free for thirty-five years now.

Greg became a teaching assistant at the piano institute, working with other injured pianists. He later got referrals for typists suffering from the same sorts of injuries. The rest is history, as Greg has employed the same techniques he learned at the piano to the computer keyboard. At this point in writing this book, my injuries flared up, so Greg taught me keystroke timing, whereby you focus your effort on the vertical dissent into the key while maintaining correct alignment and support throughout the hands and fingers. It's completely opposite to how I was taught to type, and it takes months to learn. But I don't experience any pain when practicing his technique. I'm excited about incorporating it into my regular typing.

Remember those statistics about force given earlier? Greg disputes that one standard amount of pressure goes into the typical keystroke; there is too much variation among individuals to allow for a single numerical answer. And he sees hardly any impact trauma to the fingertips. He does, however, see a lot of wrist deviation (where your hand is cocked either inward or outward) and overlifting (where your wrist bends too much up and down). He says, "That's because when you take an online typing class, that's what they tell you to do!"[6]

Greg emphasizes that he's just a field-worker. "I'm relatively uneducated about this. Don't pretend to be an expert in this field at all. But what I do know is the practical application of typing technique is something nobody's looking at."[7]

Jonathan Bailin, a trained ergonomist, emphasizes a bigger picture when evaluating how a worker performs a job. "I look at the person I'm sitting in front of, listen to what they're lifestyle is and relationship to exercise and try to get them to recognize the potency of their general physical habits on their work."[8] The worker could be someone who gets no exercise at all or who runs five miles a day. The former quite simply doesn't move enough, whereas the latter might move incorrectly at the computer.

Greg Dempster emphasizes that his retraining intervention is only appropriate in an industrial setting at a very specific moment in the course of an injury. He achieves good outcomes with people who have not yet reached the chronic stages, who've just had surgery, or whose injury has just happened. In other words, his bailiwick is the localized, garden-variety, low-grade RSI. But, Greg admits, ergonomics is not a panacea; it's preventative, not curative. And, as we've already seen in Bailin's example of the person who runs five miles a day, exercise alone is neither prevention nor cure. "The basic reason I have to show up is to look someone in the eyes and tell them your lifestyle and approach to exercise needs to change. Nothing you find on the Internet about ergonomics is going to do that," says Bailin.[9]

WHERE TO START

As medically incomplete as they might have been, the value of the way RSIs were explained to me came when I began to see my muscles were not individual structures but an interwoven amoeba of soft tissues, all working together. From that, I understood that it didn't matter where I tried to make a dent into the multiple feedback loops of RSI, so long as I could affect something somewhere along the line, because that would affect everything else in the injury. So I just jumped in. I stabbed at everything—took the spaghetti-on-the-wall approach. Since even the experts don't entirely know, I figured there is no right or wrong, unless it hurts you. I found the complexity of the disorder helps in this regard because, in a way, it doesn't matter what symptoms you can manage to alleviate; once one starts to ease, in my experience, others follow suit. Yes, every symptom you make headway with will flare up and then subside multiple times. But once you begin to make traction, you can establish a baseline and track the activities that help with or worsen your RSIs. Walking always helped me, oddly enough, even when it hurt. One day, walking three blocks would make me feel great; the next day or the next week, I'd collapse at block two, but I'd feel much better the day after that. This is to be expected. Be patient. Your musculature will fight your efforts. Be diligent. You will begin to see patterns in your RSIs, and once you do, you can start to devise larger strategies to combat them. This will feel like more than progress; you'll glimpse a light at the end of the tunnel, and it will help you get through the flare-ups and the setbacks. Once you find something that works, keep doing it. If you get discouraged in one avenue, take another that has worked. If nothing works, just rest for a time. That is doing something for your RSIs as well.

Once you begin to make some headway, you will start to feel hope. You need hope to believe you can get better; if you don't believe you can get better, you won't. That hope, in turn, renews your efforts, so that you stop seeing setbacks as setbacks. Instead, you can begin to see them as important learning experiences that actually help your overall recovery.

I did not try all the treatments that have reported success with RSIs. Some treatments I tried worked for a time, then, for varying reasons, stopped. Some treatments I tried did not work so well, affirming what I already knew: if it looks like a medieval torture device, it is in fact a medieval torture device. I found that I made more progress when undergoing two different types of treatments at once. You might not have that experience. I never had a hard time discerning the effects each treatment was having. Talk to both practitioners for a coordinated approach. Once you reach the end of the benefits of one treatment, switch to another rather than become discouraged. Choose a new treatment that addresses a different aspect of your RSIs or addresses the same one in a progressive way. What follows is a list of treatments I've tried or that have come highly recommended to me from multiple sources I trust. It is important to remember that your mileage may vary. The good news is that the online RSI community is very good about sharing resources. A number of great websites and Listservs are listed in appendix A. Do your research until you feel you can make an informed decision.

The practitioner you choose to work with is also crucial. My approach to managing my RSIs drew from many different disciplines. When faced with such a serious injury, I felt more comfortable with traditional practitioners, at least until I got a handle on listening to my own body—a very important step in the recovery process. Once I became more familiar with medical terminology and could see how the different RSI theories were working in my own injury, I began to speak to alternative practitioners. Alternative practitioners, who had strong foundations in allopathic medicine as well, gave me more confidence in trying their approach. I offer an outline of my recovery strategy also in appendix A as a guideline. It gives you an idea of the considerations involved as you approach learning to manage your RSIs.

WHAT'S AVAILABLE

Active Release Techniques (ART) is widely regarded as one of the most successful interventions for RSIs, particularly in the early stages. Developed by chiropractor P. Michael Leahy in 1985, ART is a massage technique that penetrates the scar tissue and loosens the lesions that form in soft tissues as a result of overuse. As a treatment for RSIs, ART has a 71 percent efficacy rate.[10] Recall from chapter 3 bodyworker Lamar Bush's description of the process of a muscle shortening through reciprocal inhibition. Bush explains that ART stimulates the play between the agonist and the antagonist muscles, reversing the reciprocity, so that the agonist in motion becomes the antagonist, naturally causing the other muscle to release. Let's go back to poor posture and take a muscle like the "six-pack." This key postural muscle stretches across your stomach and also plays an important role in exhaling. If your six-pack becomes substantially inhibited, it stops reciprocating with the muscles in the back, and they become unable to facilitate the activity as well as they should. And when they're unable to perform because the six-pack is chronically contracted from hours of sitting, now you're stuck like glue hunched over your computer, even when you try to sit up straight. ART helps unstick the soft tissues. Make sure any practitioner you work with has been certified by Dr. Leahy's program.

Physical and occupational therapists are also considered front-liners in the battle with RSIs. The difference between the two is that occupational therapists are trained to work with your environment and assistive tools, as well as your injury, whereas physical therapists focus more on movement. You might choose to work with an occupational therapist if, for example, a specific tool at work is giving you trouble. If your RSIs are hand centered, hand specialists in each discipline have made a particular study of the hands and the upper body, in addition to their regular training. They should be well versed in RSIs. Ask them how often they've seen patients with these injuries and what outcome you can expect. If you're suffering from thoracic outlet syndrome (TOS), make sure the practitioner you choose has worked with the Edgelow Protocol developed by physical therapist Peter Edgelow, who pioneered TOS treatments. His protocol remains the gold standard in the field.

Physical and occupational therapy are particularly nice in that you can easily measure your progress, often from week to week. Controversy has arisen over the efficacy of physical therapy for RSIs. The work-hardening approach, where muscles are strengthened through weight lifting, is not thought to be that effective. Additional downsides include that once you reach a certain range of motion, according to the health-care system, you're better and able to return to work. If you're still in pain or can't work, you'll suddenly find yourself in a gap between disciplines just when you're starting to make progress. If you need to continue exercising under professional guidance, where do you go? To a personal trainer?

There are a number of gaps in what I'll call rehabilitation workflow within our current health-care system. Filling these gaps are alternative treatments that are slowly being accepted—but not by insurance companies. I found a lot of this when transitioning from traditional health care or alternative care to the therapeutic end of recreational or sports fields. Licensing standards have yet to catch up, so you have to be careful in selecting a practitioner. This is where being educated about RSIs really comes in handy. Talk to potential practitioners; find out how many patients or clients they've seen with RSIs. Ask them to explain how their modality helps RSIs and what you should expect from treatment. Ask what kind of training they've received. Don't sign up for multiple treatments until you've tried both the modality and the practitioner a few times. Recognize that you could respond to one and not the other.

These licensing gaps are a pet peeve of mine because it really wouldn't take much to fix this problem, and we would all benefit tremendously. Let's start with massage therapy. My orthopedist prescribed this for me, recognizing the benefits it would bring, but I could not find a massage therapist able to work within the workers' compensation system. Physical therapists often give massage as part of their treatment, but they're not trained specifically as massage therapists; nor are they able to provide a full hour of massage, and that makes a big difference with a musculoskeletal injury. Massage therapists, on the other hand, have no idea how to interface with an insurance company. The lack of standardized licensing and organization within the massage profession leaves gaping holes in care.

How massage therapy became licensed in the first place is a story in itself. Thirty years ago, massage therapists apprenticed under another therapist for many years before striking out on their own. Massage therapy finally first became licensed under prostitution laws. Today, massage therapy licensing laws are a mess. Requirements vary from state to state; Wyoming, Kansas, Minnesota, and Oklahoma have no state regulation at all, whereas Nebraska, New York, and Puerto Rico require one thousand hours of training. The mean licensing requirement in the United States is five hundred hours. That's a big difference. In January 2013, the National Certification Board for Therapeutic Massage and Bodywork (NCBTMB) established a national certification in order to address these inequities. It requires 750 hours of education and 250 hours of hands-on work experience.

Therapeutic massage is very different from a spa massage. Someone who's had a hard day at the office needs a much different therapy than someone in chronic pain. I'm not belittling relaxation massage: stress is a serious health concern. But those of us requiring a more aggressive intervention should look for a therapist with a lot of training, and the national certification is a good place to start.

When a massage therapist claims to be a bodyworker, look for certifications in a variety of techniques. Specific disciplines like Reiki and Rolfing require therapists to undergo strenuous education before they can be licensed. Reiki has three levels of certification, and Rolfing has one. Most massage techniques offer some sort of certificate upon completion of training; how many a therapist has will give you an idea of the degree of his or her training and areas of interest. NCBTMB-certified massage therapist Lamar

Bush points out that good communication skills and a respectful attitude are also traits to look for in a good massage therapist. He emphasizes a third skill as well: intelligent touch, or "a perception in [the] hands to know what kind of tissue is in distress, and what kind of technique will alleviate that kind of stress in that tissue."[11]

Bush has been trained in a dozen different techniques, taught several, and even developed one or two of his own. His explanation of RSIs corresponded with what I'd already learned and was experiencing with my own injury. He works closely with a number of MDs on a regular basis, mixing holistic concepts with orthodox anatomy. All this gave me a lot of confidence that I would receive at least some benefit from trying his approach. If you apply this type of reasoning when selecting practitioners, you will also become very good at choosing the ones that will serve you best.

Bush used a combination of ART and other techniques over a three-hour session the first time, releasing many of the major muscles in my body. It was not a feel-good massage. But when I got up off his table, I remembered what it felt like to have a "normal" body. More importantly, my muscles remembered. Now they had a baseline to work with, and so did I. From there, I could chart my progress, which informed my overall treatment plan.

LISTENING TO YOUR PAIN

One of the practitioners who gave a lecture to LARSI spoke about Vipassana meditation, where you sit still and listen; it is central to the practice of mindfulness. The practitioner reported that her patients had success with using Vipassana in pain management. As I did with other practitioners, I listened with a cautious ear. Then, a friend, Kelly Carlin, called the very next day to invite me to a weekly Vipassana meditation group she was starting in her home. It was coming too easily not to give it a try.

The meditation involves sitting still for twenty minutes and attempting to clear your mind. It's okay if you have to move; just make it a part of your mindfulness practice. The meditation allows you to begin to listen to your pain, to your body, to yourself. Somehow, just listening made the pain less sharp. The more I listened, the quieter it became. Apparently it no longer had to scream to get my attention. Dr. David Williams's research at the University of Michigan Chronic Pain and Fatigue Research Center bears this out: "Pain can be modulated; you can control it or not control it, as it descends from the brain back down to the body."[12] The meditation, the listening, slows or dampens the pain information as it travels. Pain is trying to tell you something, and if you listen to it, you can at least temper it.

Acupuncture also reports a lot of success in treating RSIs, and it, too, has undergone a tremendous shift in licensing. To become an acupuncturist in

China, you must first go to medical school and then to a four-year college of acupuncture. Acupuncturists in the United States are now required to attend a three- or four-year, graduate-level, accredited program to be licensed. Most insurance in the United States now covers acupuncture as well.

When it came to selecting a practitioner, I choose one who had been a surgeon in Moscow, then studied acupuncture with a Chinese master before coming to the United States. She put twenty-five needles in my neck, back, arms, and sometimes even my feet. She put electrical stimulation on the needles and left me on the table for an hour. Acupuncture stimulates the body's natural opiates and opens up its energy centers, according to the Chinese system, encouraging its own natural healing.

Once I'd received a short number of treatments, my body craved them. As soon as I hit the table, even before she put in the needles, I fell asleep. Next thing I knew, I was waking up from the most delicious slumber. I got more rest on that table than I had since becoming injured. Deep rest and relaxation may not sound like much, but when you're suffering from a stress injury, they are key to rehabilitation. With deep rest, your body is able to repair itself. Deep relaxation begins to take hold outside the treatments, your muscles begin to relax, the pain lessens, and functionality slowly begins to return.

LEARNING TO MOVE AGAIN

Yoga is another modality with serious licensing challenges. There are a number of different types of yoga, with teaching certification varying for each type. Some swear by Bikram yoga, especially for the back. I watched a class once and laughed; there was no way I could do any of that. Once again, LARSI offered some help navigating this world when senior intermediate Level II Iyengar instructor Anna Delury came to talk to the group. I had tried yoga before, but when the teacher asked me to do a handstand, I knew I could not put that much weight on my wrists and refused. The teacher thought I was babying my wrists. I left the class and stand by my decision. No practitioner should ask you to do something that will hurt you. At the same time, practitioners won't know what will hurt you unless you tell them. If you do so and the practitioner doesn't back off, go elsewhere. That's a good sign he or she knows nothing about RSIs.

At the support group meeting that day, Anna asked us to kneel on our feet on the floor, and I couldn't even do that. As I was struggling, she glanced over and suggested an adjustment that allowed me to get into the pose. I trusted her after that.

I believe there are only two reasons why I was able to study yoga: first, it was Iyengar and not another type, and second, Anna was my teacher. Iyengar yoga is very precise. You get into a pose and hold it. There's not a lot of movement. It develops strength, alignment, stability, balance, and endurance. Other systems of yoga do not focus so much on alignment, and if you are already suffering from poor alignment, as anyone with RSIs is, the result is a house of cards. The teacher is crucial to learning yoga. I was extremely lucky to have found a teacher like Anna because she is well known in therapeutics, having studied directly under B. K. S. Iyengar himself for many, many years. In fact, Anna also trains Iyengar teachers in Los Angeles, many of whom specifically come to study therapeutics with her. There were often two or three teachers in the class, learning from Anna as she taught her students. If I complained about my back or elbows, Anna would put me in a pose, make any adjustments, explain to me what she was trying to do, and then turn to the teaching students who had gathered around and explain even more to them. I learned so much.

Anna described RSIs as "this computer stuff," using the image of a tangled necklace and how you have to roll the chain back and forth to work out the knots. That image sure mimicked my experience. When I first came to her class, I couldn't do downward-facing dog. She had me put my hands on the seat of a chair to do the pose. That stretched my back out wonderfully, so I could get at least some benefits from the pose. The use of props is also a hallmark of Iyengar yoga. You can't work toward a pose if you never develop what's necessary to get into it in the first place. To this day, this method of using props and easing partially into a new exercise allows me to continue to rehabilitate my body. It took a year and a half before I could do downward-facing dog with my hands on the floor. I've studied yoga now for six years, and I still can't hold the pose for very long, but the MD and the physical therapist on my health-care team are both astounded that I can do it at all.

"What you learned from Anna had to do with you,"[13] says Dr. Marian Garfinkel, also a senior intermediate Iyengar instructor. Dr. Garfinkel has conducted a scientific study on Iyengar yoga and carpal tunnel syndrome, publishing it in the peer-reviewed *Journal of the American Medical Association*. Now this is a carpal tunnel study. It compares wrist splints to Iyengar yoga, two very different treatments, but the results are telling. The yoga group saw significant improvement in grip strength and a significant reduction in pain, whereas the control group saw no significant changes in grip strength and pain.[14] I would say that's evidence enough that when your doctor prescribes wrist braces, you may want to check out your local Iyengar yoga center.

Dr. Garfinkel has also studied directly with B. K. S. Iyengar, attending every intensive seminar he has taught since 1975. She says that when studying yoga, "you have to practice, and you have to have a good teacher, one who knows what they're talking about."[15] About teachers she says, "Lots of people are getting certified to teach; the sad part is that they want to teach right away. In Iyengar yoga, it doesn't work that way. You can get certified in other types of yoga quickly, but it's not the same."[16] In my experience, the Iyengar system is extremely good not only for RSIs but for back pain. Again, the key is using props and having a good teacher who knows how to work with your body to allow it to get into poses.

Another movement modality I studied was Feldenkreis. In this instance, the Multiple Sclerosis Society vetted an instructor for me. The society held a class at my local library, and, frankly, it was a bit weird. Feldenkreis uses a somatic technique, working in micro-movements to trigger your brain to remember how to perform that movement correctly. We'd work on one specific part of the body in each class, lifting our right shoulder toward the ceiling, releasing it down on the floor, lifting it toward the ceiling again. For an hour. At the start of every class, we performed a body scan to see how we were standing, what felt tight, sore, and stiff, how our limbs hung at our sides, if we were listing, how our pelvis sat, how our feet were planted on the floor. At the end of class, when we scanned our bodies again, I always noticed a difference. Pretty quickly, I began to see that I was walking differently, sitting differently, and moving differently.

In yoga, they talk about "the edge," the limit of what your body can do at any given time. Learning to work with the edge helps tremendously with RSIs. You learn to feel for it, listen for it, and recognize it; then you can decide if you want to push yourself a little or your body is telling you to take it easy. I was sent to a cognitive behavioral therapist for the sleep disorder I had developed due to my injury. She gave me a great tip: stop when you feel like you can still do more. That way, you come away from a task feeling confident and satisfied that you were able to do it rather than frustrated because you'll never be able to do it. Such a small thing can have a huge impact.

Part 2

THE POLITICS OF RSIs

Chapter Six

Why the Health-Care Community Disputes the Existence of RSIs

The health-care community has been late to the party when it comes to repetitive strain injuries. Despite all the clinical evidence, there is still tremendous controversy over what RSIs are and whether they exist at all. How can this be? Doctors say there is insufficient medical evidence that any insult to tissue occurs through repetitive motion, employers say they're not work related, insurance companies use both arguments to avoid paying for them, and the pharmaceutical industry ignores them as there's no money to be made. Doctors had gotten around the problem of so many patients presenting with complaints versus the lack of medical evidence by creating a set of clinical diagnoses, categorizations of the disorders based on the sheer amount of corroborative anecdotal evidence, but the symptoms, diagnostics, and treatments all remain contentious twenty years after the epidemic first took hold. Even though RSIs remain the number one occupational illness in the country and are the most common cause of physical disability in the world,[1] very little is known about them. And I say incredibly powerful forces have a huge financial stake in keeping it that way.

For instance, Dr. Barry Simmons, chief of the Hand and Upper Extremity Service in the Department of Orthopedic Surgery at Boston's Brigham and Women's Hospital, makes the whole thing sound so simple: "In the scientific community, who deals with upper-extremity disorders, it's accepted that keyboard use does not cause carpal tunnel syndrome," says Simmons.[2] This sounds like a definitive dismissal of the entire subject—except that there is a proven correlation between upper-extremity pain and computer usage, just not carpal tunnel syndrome specifically with keyboard usage. Epidemiologist Judith Gold carefully chooses her words when she agrees with Dr. Simmons, stipulating that we can't say "cause," because we don't know for sure that there is a correlation. Gold states emphatically, "RSIs are real."[3] In other words, the existence of certain symptoms as being caused by certain technological tools has yet to be proven or disproven, but statistical relationships have been proven to exist between certain symptoms and certain tools, tasks, or jobs. Everything else that I present in the remainder of this book turns on this fact alone: there is a mincing of words here, words that mean one thing to a scientist and something else entirely to the public. There are those who are interested in disproving that computers cause injury, for example, or that truck driving damages the back; others, such as unions, are interested in proving this, each for obvious reasons. Everyone has an opinion, and all stakeholders are passionate about their position. I believe a number of powerful economic forces are at play here. This is the crux of RSIs as an economic, political, and social problem.

Definitive "medical evidence" comes from research data period. Research is an expensive game controlled by big pharmaceutical companies. There is plenty of clinical data, but it has yet to be assembled comprehensively for two reasons: first, the little guys in the field are swamped by an epidemic and not organized; second, the patchwork quilt of disorders, diagnostics, and definitions assembled in the midst of the epidemic has made a mess of an already complex set of syndromes. To straighten this mess out, we almost have to go back to square one.

LACK OF TRAINING

When I was a kid, whatever the doctor said, my mother did religiously. People saw doctors as godlike, a view promulgated by advancements in medicine. I mean, they transplanted a heart, for Pete's sake; they sure seemed like gods. But they weren't. They were and are amazing, but medical doctors are not infallible. Medical school does not give them every bit of knowledge they need to practice medicine. It gives them a good foundation, but they're expected to gain more from their residency in their specialty and even more from continuing education once they begin to practice. There is a vast amount of knowledge in the field, and for all its science, it turns out, the practice of medicine is still an art.

Medical doctors are trained to treat acute injury and disease; RSI is neither. Pain—what causes it, its processes, and its treatments—is not taught in medical school, even though, logically, it's the biggest reason why patients go to the doctor in the first place. Pain is usually taught at the residency level, generally to specialists like anesthesiologists and rheumatologists. So, typical general practitioners or internists do not learn about pain unless they take a continuing medical education course on the subject. This education often comes through the system of medical journals, which, it turns out, are little fiefdoms of information. RSIs, for example, cannot be written about in the family practice journal because they are the domain of the pain management journal. So if the pain management journal doesn't have the editorial space to cover RSIs because, say, prescription drug abuse is considered a more important topic, family practitioners do not receive the information about RSIs.

Nor have family practitioners likely received much training in RSI, according to a 2007 study by the American Academy of Orthopedic Surgeons (AAOS). As part of its "US Bone and Joint Decade" campaign, the AAOS set out to improve the musculoskeletal knowledge of primary care physicians because they're the ones who actually see the most patients with musculoskeletal conditions. Even though musculoskeletal conditions account for 10 to 28 percent of all primary care visits, most primary care physicians don't feel comfortable with their level of knowledge about them.[4] The AAOS survey of family practice physicians found 51 percent felt that they had insufficient training in orthopedics, and 56 percent said that medical school was their only source for formal musculoskeletal training. The survey also reported that only 51 of the 122 medical schools in the United States have a dedicated musculoskeletal course; only 25 schools require a course in musculoskeletal medicine, either in rheumatology, orthopedics, or physical medicine and rehabilitation; and nearly half of all medical schools in the United States (57) don't require any musculoskeletal course at all.[5]

The AAOS has set out to change that, but Dr. George Piligian, assistant professor of preventive medicine at Mount Sinai School of Medicine in New York, thinks medical training should go one step further. He primarily teaches how to look for clues to disease, to determine causative factors, and to apply this information in treatment. "I think this is the way all of medical treatment should be structured."[6] Piligian says one of the obstacles in the way of optimizing RSI treatment is that practitioners may not have the ability to incorporate the fruits of the best research on RSIs into their clinical practice. He says there's a need for consensus in the scientific community among those who study RSIs in order to provide better guidance for medical practitioners.

Piligian believes that at the heart of achieving that consensus is redefining RSIs. He describes them as a process that needs to be discussed among practitioners and researchers in order to come up with a definitive definition. Piligian would call an RSI "a threshold in which the patient is aware of discomfort in a specific body part, that can be manifested in a number of ways, such as numbness, pain, awareness of the body part, abnormal sensations, or functional impairments, such as loss of endurance in muscle function. Eventually the process can result in functional impairment."[7]

Another reason RSIs remain so controversial is that the diagnosis is clinical, not pathological. Because the scientific evidence was not available in the face of an epidemic, clinic evidence became the basis for diagnosis. However, unless and until a pathological diagnosis is found, the controversy cannot be settled. Dr. James D. Collins at UCLA, a rock star radiologist, has found that pathological diagnosis. Collins says that clinical diagnostics reflect confounding training in and misunderstanding of RSIs. "Doctors are missing the diagnoses because their assistant often takes the blood pressure and does not report the patient's complaints while their blood pressure is being taken."[8] Collins says the pathology is simple: the patient has decreased blood flow in the arterial return from the heart to the brain because of impediment in the venous return. "All you have to do is put a blood pressure cuff on a thoracic outlet syndrome patient and have the patient stand up. They'll pass out because of decreased blood supply," says Collins.[9]

Collins shares some other truly imaginative testing techniques developed by colleagues that demonstrate both what's possible and what's lacking in diagnostics. Dr. David Agnew in Santa Barbara, California, takes the blood pressure measurement on both arms while the patient is seated, first with the arms down and then again when they're up. Dr. Ernestina Saxton in Fresno, California, takes incremental blood pressure measurements. Dr. Richard Braun in San Diego puts the patient's hand in water and measures the displacement. To trigger complaints, Dr. Braun raises the patient's arm overhead before repeating the test and looking for changes in water displacement. Dr. Braun also places a pulse oximeter on each of the patient's fingers. But the diagnostic problem that really gets Dr. Collins's goat is the new disposable blood pressure cuffs. Their bladders exist in only a small section of the plastic cuff that wraps around the entire arm, so the pressure applied is uneven around the circumference. How can you get accurate circulatory information from that?

LACK OF DEFINITIVE DIAGNOSTICS

The nerve-conduction study has been the go-to diagnostic for carpal tunnel syndrome since 1956, except many who report all the symptoms of carpal tunnel syndrome register either a false negative or a false positive because of a lack of standardized diagnostic criteria. A whopping 16 to 34 percent of clinically defined carpal tunnel syndrome is being misdiagnosed via the nerve-conduction study.[10] Inconsistencies in the method of examination and interpretation of results make the other two most popular tests, Phalen's and Tinel's, unreliable as well. Plus, all of these test for carpal tunnel syndrome. What if you have radial tunnel syndrome or Guyon's tunnel syndrome or any of the other RSIs? Collins again states, "With these tests, all you're doing is looking at the blood supply." Upon first examination, though, these are the three tests recommended by the American Medical Association. If the findings don't come cleanly and conclusively on all three tests, the patient's diagnosis is ambiguous. This is where the arguing begins.

Only a pathological diagnosis can stop the arguing. Dr. Collins's research has provided that pathology: "It's all vascular."[11] In 1983, while teaching anatomy at UCLA, Dr. Collins was presented with an MRI machine that would display three-dimensional images. "Nobody wanted anything to do with it. I thought it was another gimmick."[12] But with the 3D MRA/MRV, Collins could see landmark anatomy never seen before. Using a process called phase encoding, he could generate a color-coded image that visually distinguished blood vessels from and within the nerves, from and within the muscles, and from and within the lymph system. Suddenly, everything became much clearer. Collins could see pathologies that had not been displayed before.

The 3D MRA/MRV machine revealed important findings: first, nerves have a bloody supply; second, veins have bicuspid valves. He discovered the first by imaging an artery with the machine programmed to color-code nerves as well; the resultant image revealed that nerves bind to arteries for their nutrient blood supply. Collins's research also displayed that compressing a nerve also compresses its blood supply. Now Collins could see that in action. He displayed that, with TOS, loose, untoned muscles in the shoulder cause compression of the valves in the veins of the neck, preventing the blood from draining properly.

The second finding is important because it means to me that you need the right amount of muscle tone throughout your body for venous return. Insufficient compression prevents the circulatory system from working correctly. Dr. Collins' pathological diagnosis for RSIs then is costoclavicular compression. If it is not corrected, tissue degenerates not just in the brachial plexus but also in the brain because the blood is not draining properly from your head. This causes short-term memory loss, headaches, and TMJ, among other things often associated with RSI.

Collins findings reveal that migraine, carpal tunnel syndrome, reflex sympathetic dystrophy syndrome, dystonia, fibromyalgia, impingement, piriformis syndrome, and thoracic outlet syndrome are all due to a decrease in blood flow. The assumption, up until now, has been that RSIs are caused by changes in the fascia because pain, it is known, is caused by expansion of the facial plane. Dr. Collins's research displays that the expansion is coming from backed up blood vessels pressing against the fascia, and that relationship should be the point of reference, not the fascia itself. "The pain these patients experience comes from the veins backing up because the blood can't get out," he says.[13] What this means for treatment, however, is a whole other matter, and Collins has an uphill battle with doctors—other than those who send him patients, of course. Early on, he began annotating patients' images for their doctors' review because they didn't know enough about anatomy.

Those doctors could then call him to discuss his findings. He also incorporates his studies when training new doctors, nurses, and other health professionals, and in this way, the information gets disseminated, albeit slowly. Similar research in vascular compromise has popped up in a Spanish study involving the effects of vibrations on workers' upper extremities.[14] But these results have yet to affect treatment at the clinical level.

Looking at the circulatory system is just one aspect of the latest research in RSIs. The common diagnosis of tendonitis is also getting a revision. Tendonitis means inflammation of the tendon. Yet biopsies of tendonitis sites did not show an inflammatory process. Instead, they showed a combination of degeneration and incomplete regeneration of the tissues. "What regenerates is not able to make up for what's degenerated," says Dr. Piligian. That's because veins don't regenerate; they divert. According to Piligian, "This represents a huge paradigm shift."[15] Tendonitis should now be called tendinosis, but clinical practice has not yet caught up with the name change.

These pathological findings still present problems. As health professionals use science to prove and disprove the existence of RSIs, those who suffer from them applaud all these pioneering efforts, even as their own battles remain frustrating. So many cases have been denied for lack of evidence when the evidence is there, but the insurance company won't pay for the test, or the radiologist doesn't know how to read the images, or the doctor reading the radiologist's report doesn't know enough about anatomy. Dr. Collins and others have argued with all of these various individuals. One TOS patient had to take her case all the way to US district court to continue receiving disability benefits. She had to fight the American Medical Association's treatment guidelines, which, shockingly, are based on all this incomplete knowledge. Collins interjects, "How can you make guidelines for something you know nothing about?"[16] Well, it happens all the time, I'm sure, because something has to be done while we are waiting for the science to catch up. But enough is enough.

Clinical diagnoses alone are not allowed to form the basis for either treatment guidelines or diagnostic codes, the classifying system for all disorders and treatments used throughout the health-care system. When only clinical evidence is available, or when large sections of the scientific community dispute pathological evidence, there is much room for argument. The result is a very cautious compromise. In the case of RSIs, caution often results in futile treatment, and revising both diagnostic codes and treatment guidelines involves a lengthy, often political process. If the diagnostic code for a particular disorder does not include the most recent research or takes into account clinical evidence only, then the entire health-care system must continue to rely on outdated treatment protocols, even after they have been proven wrong. For a patient, this can mean a life in ruins.

Collins's vascular theory means that surgery for TOS is still possible, but the right physical therapy protocols for TOS should be done before and after surgery. Collins suggests that physical therapy be ongoing for the rest of the patient's life! From a legal perspective, that is never something an insurance company wants to hear. Dr. Piligian, who is in the trenches with his patients, grounds the missing science in a practical way: "What's available has not caught up with what's going on with people's bodies, so that leaves a lot of leeway for those who care for injured workers and for those whose job it is to adjudicate whether the disability or an impairment are warranted and should be compensated."[17]

Many of us have heard of the *Diagnostic and Statistical Manual of Mental Disorders* (*DSM*) due to a controversial recent update in the news particularly affecting autism. If you've been following the process of updating the autism definition in the *DSM*, you see just how difficult it is to get the diagnostic code for any disease changed. Now let's apply that to the human level, where those of us suffering from an injury or ailment have to survive. At the time of my injury, the diagnostic code for carpal tunnel syndrome called for twenty-one days off work, rest, wrist bracing, and/or surgery, and so that was all the insurance company was willing to authorize. Time off and rest didn't work, and because I also had bilateral radial tunnel syndrome and TOS, surgery on my carpal tunnels would not have alleviated my symptoms. Yet this was the only treatment available to me without a fight. In my case, it was a five-year fight that actually worsened my RSI instead of making it better.

SURGICAL OUTCOMES

Even as it wages war over whether RSIs exist, big health care has also rushed in to make sure it can profit from them. Carpal tunnel surgery has become big business. The *New York Times* reports that more than half a million Americans undergo surgery for carpal tunnel syndrome annually. Yet, carpal tunnel surgery in the RSI community has a very bad reputation for a variety of reasons, including residual pain, poor return-to-work outcomes, residual scar tissue exacerbating the underlying neuromuscular problems, and out-and-out misdiagnosis.

Kevin C. Chung's 2006 review of carpal tunnel surgery efficacy for the journal *Hand* reveals that although there is improvement after surgery, patients still report pain, and functional improvements are only modest. It's important to point out here that reduction in pain alone is nice, but if you can't use your hands, you're effectively left disabled. A study of the Canadian health-care system found that four years after their surgeries, 46 percent of patients had moderate to severe pain, and 52 percent had moderate to severe numbness. While 64 percent of the study subjects returned to the same job, only 14 percent were symptom-free. The American Academy of Orthopaedic Surgeons' own guidelines read, "We do not have sufficient evidence to provide specific treatment recommendations for carpal tunnel syndrome when found in association with . . . the workplace."[18]

The New York State Workers' Compensation Board's guidelines for treatment of carpal tunnel syndrome state, "The concept of 'cure' with respect to surgical treatment by itself is generally a misnomer."[19] It should be noted, in the workers' compensation system's defense, that it is only required to return patients to work, if possible, not to life as they knew it before their injuries. This is an extremely important point for workers to remember.

EROSION OF TRUST

All this has eroded trust between health-care providers and patients, regardless of what ails them. And this erosion, coupled with the 15.4 percent of Americans who are uninsured, is creating massive public health issues as more and more people simply do not go to the doctor.[20] Patients are every bit as much the problem in the health-care system as the practitioners and institutions. Because we hate "the doctor," many of us have stopped going, and so the doctor can't prevent the diseases they are so good at detecting. It is where all the research dollars have been spent, and that is a good thing. So go to the doctor regularly, but go as a partner in your health care. Don't wait for Washington to change the system; interact with the system differently. Doing so is the prerogative not only of the wealthy and the educated but also of employers who want to cut down on their health-care costs and insurance companies who cannot sustain their business models.

And if your doctor treats you like you're crazy, challenge him about the classes he did and did not take in medical school.

Chapter Seven

How the Workers' Compensation System Worsens RSIs

In the United States, 69.4 percent of repetitive strain injury cases are attributed to work.[1] If you contract an RSI at work, you will have to file a workers' compensation claim; if you later discover your RSI is not work related, your regular health insurance may not cover it. So if you are at risk for RSIs, you should know some very important things about the American workers' compensation system before you find yourself at its mercy.

A group of corporate lawyers devised the US workers' compensation system in the early part of the twentieth century—right around the time J. P. Morgan formed US Steel and big business was born. The advent of megacorporations engendered a slew of new legal issues, one of the most difficult being injured workers. Costs were hard to predict, presenting a problem when it came time to calculate dividends and whatnot. At the time, a worker had to file a lawsuit against his or her employer in order to recover damages from an injury, requiring money to hire lawyers, which most injured workers did not have. Employers, on the other hand, who had plenty of money, could use what was called the "unholy trinity" of defenses by asserting that the worker was in some way responsible for his injury; that a fellow worker, not the employer, was responsible for the injury; or that the employee knew the job was hazardous and, by agreeing to work, assumed those risks. These cases could be tied up in court for years.

In the era of manufacturing, many more workers were getting injured, and popular sentiment decried the injustice; legally, however, it was a state matter. Congress did try to weigh in, and President William Howard Taft drew on interstate commerce laws to protect transportation workers; still, most Americans were unprotected. Eventually a team of lawyers stepped in, ostensibly to help workers, when, in fact, they were really out to solve the accounting problem. They devised what has become the workers' compensation system.[2] The system was adopted via legislation on a state-by-state basis, with very little public debate. The American people never got a chance to vote on it.

THE SYSTEM VIOLATES WORKERS' CONSTITUTIONAL RIGHTS

With implementation of this system, workers were made to give up their right to due process, something we give criminals every day, when the lawyers got rid of jury trials. The accountants wanted to be able to predict how much money work-related injuries were going to cost, so they created a schedule of payments according to severity of the injury. In addition, treatment guidelines, a fairly recent addition to the system, today place control of the injured workers' health care in the hands of system-selected panels, not doctors. The fees lawyers could charge to represent workers were significantly reduced to decrease litigation costs for injured workers, except these fees are based upon a percentage of the workers' final award, so the only ones to save money were the insurance companies. It also makes most of that representation inadequate because the better lawyers go for the higher-paying areas of practice. Workers' compensation lawyers fall far below ambulance chasers in terms of percentage collected. After a few tries, workers' compensation lawyers did manage to debunk the unholy trinity, especially the one about assumed risk. It was touted as a victory for workers at the time, when really it was a circumvention of the US constitution from the start.

As bad as it was at inception, once insurance companies stepped in to provide coverage for employers and the system played out, major problems became immediately apparent: the injured worker, as the plaintiff, must prove that she's been injured on the job, just like anyone suing anyone else in this country—except, in the workers' compensation system, you have to use a doctor approved by the insurance company to do this, a doctor with an inherent conflict of interest. And there's another catch. The insurance company owes a duty to its policyholder to act in "good faith." With every other type of insurance, you are the policyholder, and you have leverage against the insurance company if it's not doing what it said it would do when it sold you the policy. You can take it to court, and insurance companies tend not to do very well in front of juries.

In the workers' compensation system, however, the insurance companies don't have a duty to act in good faith in the interests of the injured worker; they owe that to the employer because the employer is the policyholder. And because the system eliminated jury trials, you cannot take an insurance company to court if it is acting in bad faith. To make matters worse, employers have a strong incentive to deny workers' injuries; otherwise, their premiums will go up. Finally, because the attorneys who represent workers can only get paid so much, they can't afford to spend much time on each case. In sum: When your claim is investigated, the insurance company asks your boss if you got hurt on the job. If your boss says no, the insurance company denies the claim, forcing the injured worker to take the case to court. It's a tactic insurance companies call "starving you out." They figure if you're not receiving any compensation, you'll soon go back to work—which they then claim proves that you were never injured in the first place. Litigation almost always ensues, creating a tremendous backlog in the system that was supposed to reduce litigation, with everybody getting paid except the injured worker and the employer. In nearly 90 percent of workers' compensation litigation, the injured worker eventually wins.[3]

The system itself is supposed to penalize insurance companies for using these tactics, but, as we shall see, that doesn't happen enough to prevent an extraordinary amount of bad faith on the part of insurance companies. People accused of crimes, in fact, have more rights in this country than do injured workers, which places them below criminals on the social scale. In the criminal justice system, the accuser must prove the accused's guilt; the accused merely has to establish reasonable doubt in the minds of a jury of his or her peers. This system of checks and balances gives neither side an advantage over the other.

In the workers' compensation system, the insurance company has all the advantages, and the injured worker has none. The insurance company need prove nothing; the injured worker has to prove beyond all doubt, not just reasonable, that a work-related injury exists and that the insurance company should pay for needed treatment, using the company's own witnesses. The deck is stacked. What's more, if the insurance company loses, the employer pays the price because employers pay for the system. This means that we all do, because employers pass the cost on in the form of higher sales prices, reduced hiring, lower wages, and so on.

While litigation proceeds, the injured worker often doesn't get treatment or receive disability benefits, or the practitioner treating the injured worker doesn't get paid, resulting in a high number of patients per practitioner and much poorer outcomes. Add RSIs into the mix, and you have a nightmare. The California Workers' Compensation Institute's "Injury Scorecard" reports that a carpal tunnel claimant remains in the workers' compensation system for an average of just under four years, nearly triple the period for all other work-injury claims.[4] We already know RSIs worsen with delays and inadequate or incorrect treatment, so, unsurprisingly, "more than half of the carpal tunnel claims over the past decade have resulted in permanent disability—nearly triple that for all other claims."[5]

New York State's system does no better. An overhaul in 2007 increased the maximum weekly benefits, but injured workers gave up any lifetime benefits in the process. RSI cases in New York are almost always litigated before approval for treatment can begin. Cathy Stanton, head of the workers' compensation department at the law firm of Pasternack, Tilker, Ziegler, Walsh, Stanton & Romano, member of the Society of New York Workers' Compensation Bar Association, and current president of the Workers Injury Law and Advocacy Group, says that 98 percent of the RSI cases her office handles get approved after litigation, but that takes six to nine months.[6] Considering Greg Dempster's results with early intervention, the New York system is set up to worsen RSIs.

Once the RSI sufferer in New York does get his case approved, the treatment guidelines—designed for mild, garden-variety conditions—include four to five treatments of physical therapy, two to four treatments of acupuncture, six weeks of massage, and four paraffin bath treatments.[7] The New York guidelines also provide that "continuation of normal daily activities is an accepted and well-established recommendation for [carpal tunnel syndrome]."[8] The New York State Workers' Compensation Board is "reimagining" the state's workers' compensation system with a real opportunity to spearhead true cost savings.[9]

WHERE THE FRAUD REALLY IS

Injured workers who refuse the treatment prescribed by the system or who don't respond to that treatment are either forced back to work too soon or become embroiled in a legal battle that costs a tremendous amount of money and likely these patients' ability to work for a very long time, if not the rest of their lives. This is how RSIs have become the number one disability in the world, which is a shame because they needn't become disabling at all.

The ironic thing about accusing RSI patients of malingering is that they are in fact usually the hardest working people on any given staff. That's how they got injured in the first place. Every RSI patient I've ever met has been a type A personality. We're workaholics. It is also interesting to note that in every recent workers' compensation reform, maximum weekly benefits have risen, whereas wages in this country remain stagnant. This suggests that the increases are needed to cover the growing number of higher-earning RSI sufferers. In January 2012, the latest data available, nationally, maximum weekly benefits ranged from $437 in Mississippi to $1,457 in Iowa.[10] The latter covers two-thirds of an $113,646 annual salary.

When you tell someone you've filed a claim, the response is often, "Everyone who files a workers' compensation claim is faking it." That's logically impossible. We've all seen news reports of the man with the bad back waterskiing, so obviously there is some fraud. Still, even the workers' compensation insurance industry maintains that 30 percent of all claims are fraudulent.[11] This misconception derives from advertising campaigns such as that waged by one company, the Fremont Compensation Insurance Group, which, according to an article in the *Los Angeles Times*, "marketed itself as a company that could save employers money by rooting out worker and doctor fraud. It advertised on more than 600 billboards around the state that showed cheating workers behind bars. Its slogan was 'Fraud Doesn't Work Here.'"[12]

An independent team of experts during this same time found nationally that fraudulent workers' compensation claims equaled about 2 percent of total workers' compensation dollars.[13] Regardless of which statistic is correct, the actual cost of this fraud is relatively low compared to the other fraud going on in the system. According the *Los Angeles Times* article cited above, the same company that put up those six hundred billboards was later found to be committing fraud itself.[14] In fact, a 1998 audit of the California workers' compensation system revealed that insurance companies committed fraud in 120 percent of the claims audited.[15]

Arnold Schwarzenegger found himself on this battleground when he became governor of California in 2003. The California Department of Insurance was forced to take over thirty-one carriers between 1997 and 2006, and the state-run carrier, the State Compensation Insurance Fund (SCIF), at one point was underwriting over 50 percent of all policies in the state.[16] Something clearly had to be done. Except Schwarzenegger failed to address the research into the reason for these takeovers: the insurance companies were underestimating claims and failing to set aside the proper reserves. The Rand Corporation contends in its latest evaluation of the California system that this condition still exists.[17] I look at the statistics on the number of RSI cases in the system, how long it takes to resolve them, and how often they end in a permanent disability, and I wonder if this isn't where all of the underestimating of claims is taking place.

In the insurance industry's defense, Jeff Teideman, loss-control consultant for California's State Compensation Insurance Fund, says, "We saw just a cataclysm of carpal tunnel syndrome in the 1990s."[18] Also, around the time SCIF was underwriting so many policies, Teideman says the cataclysm caught SCIF by surprise because there was no scientific correlation between the amount of repetitive motion and the injury. The fund was studying the movement patterns looking for causation and concluded that some causation had to be happening away from the job. It continues to await research data proving its hypothesis. In the meantime, Teideman says, "there were lots of misdiagnoses. A lot of people got surgery who didn't have carpal tunnel."[19] Now, SCIF focuses more on prevention. Teideman admits, the incidents are down, but costs remain the same. In other words, fewer people are getting injured, but injuries are costing more per case. At least SCIF's efforts at prevention are effective.

Statistics released by the California Department of Workers' Compensation Audit and Enforcement Unit in 2011 shows that reforms Schwarzenegger enacted in 2003 didn't save a dime. Penalties against insurance companies seven years later ($1.4 million) are just below their 2002 levels ($2 million),[20] even though Schwarzenegger discontinued many of the penalties that could be assessed against an insurer. So although these numbers, at first glance, seem to indicate improvement, they in fact indicate more fraud on the part of insurers, not less, because there are fewer incidents for which an insurer can get penalized. The average amount of unpaid compensation per claim audited in 2011 was $1,458, and 89.6 percent of those payments were for disability benefits.[21]

A report by the Workers Injury Law and Advocacy Group says that insurance industry and employer fraud is the real problem in terms of costs and loss of revenue to society.[22] The largest source of employer fraud comes from underreporting, such as misclassifying a job as one that is less dangerous. Insurance giant AIG and its affiliated workers' compensation insurers doubled down on all the fraud by underreporting what their employer customers were paying in workers' compensation premiums. AIG was fined $100 million, plus $46.5 million in taxes, in 2010 for misreporting $2.12 billion as general or commercial liability premiums instead of workers' compensation premiums.[23]

The National Insurance Crime Bureau (NICB), a private-sector law enforcement agency funded by the insurance industry, aggressively tracks fraud committed by employees. Yet when former NICB vice president Jim Spiller was asked if the NICB investigated insurance companies that were ripping off consumers, he replied, "No . . . that would be a job for state insurance regulators."[24] Those regulators are established and paid for by the same workers' compensation system they are supposed to investigate. Little wonder they are underfunded and limited in the scope of what they can do.

RSI OUTCOMES IN SELF-INSURED COMPANIES

When you compare RSI outcomes among the private insurance carriers with those of self-insured companies, the differences are stark. Employers pay almost entirely for the workers' compensation system in this country—shelling out $77.1 billion in 2011—so it's no surprise that those who can afford to do so opt to fund and administer their own workers' compensation. Self-insured companies have enough capital to finance their own in-house workers' compensation systems. They set a calculated amount of money aside to pay for potential future claims and treatments. These reserves are strictly controlled by a state's department of insurance. The companies then administrate those programs themselves or hire a third-party administrator to do the work for them. In 2011, private carriers reported 57.1 percent of the total benefits they paid out were for medical costs, whereas self-insureds' medical costs comprised only 25.5 percent of their total benefits paid out. This data suggests that self-insureds are spending less on health care. But when you look at all the possible expenses in an injured worker's case—health care, temporary and permanent disability benefits, and litigation and administrative costs—a different picture begins to emerge. More of self-insureds' money is going toward benefits for injured workers. Another statistic sheds further light: employer costs for private insurers are 59.2 percent; costs for self-insureds are only 21.9 percent—less than half. Clearly, self-insured companies' administrative costs are lower as well, which means they're either providing less treatment or their treatment is more effective. It's no wonder that in 1962 only 13 percent of employers were self-insured, but by 2011 that number had nearly doubled to 23.9 percent.

A key difference is that self-insured companies receive direct information about how their safety and treatment programs are working and so are able to self-correct. Companies that pay for workers' compensation insurance rely on the insurance company to give them that information. Too often it comes in the form of claims filed, followed by a hike in premiums.

The movement-retraining field expert from chapter 5, Greg Dempster, who works mainly with self-insured companies, provides some insight: "Self-insured companies already know how much an RSI case is going to cost them. They know that getting their worker back on the job is going to cost them a lot less money."[25] Unfortunately, early-intervention and retraining approaches like Dempster's just aren't that common; the idea is still very new. "There are only 3 or 4 people in the country who are retraining computer operators. I'm the one who's probably been doing it the longest, but I've only published 3 or 4 papers."[26]

Still, intrigued by Dempster's method, Lawrence Livermore National Laboratory conducted a study on Dempster's work. Of the eighty of Dempster's clients the lab studied, 80 percent had returned to work with little to no recurrence.[27] But Dempster has been able to handpick his clients. When someone is severely injured or the injury has gone on for too long, there's not much he can do. Dempster started out thinking his method was a cure, then found that getting RSI suffers back to work successfully involves a more complex set of factors. Still, he reports that when an employer calls him in to help with a worker injury and all parties are cooperating, there's a really good chance he can achieve the employee's successful return to work. The difference? "Everybody in the circle of care understands what it's going to take to make this work," says Dempster, "and they see that it gets done."[28] He achieves a better than 80 percent return of workers' previous capacity simply because of employer cooperation.

This approach contrasts starkly with how my own case was handled. The workers' compensation insurance company kept sending me to more and more doctors, each time hoping that the new doctor would provide a more favorable evaluation of my injuries. However, because the company's doctors were so backed up and it often took six to nine months to get an appointment, I wound up developing more and more end-stage complications due to the delays. Eventually, the insurance carrier just gave up, but I'm quite certain that if my employers had been aware of how my claim was being handled, they would have opted for far less litigation and far fewer doctors on the payroll. I believe a more enlightened approach to RSI claims management is called for.

Chapter Eight

The Political Battle over RSIs

The politics of repetitive strain injuries starts with the medical establishment not wanting to give up its power or its ground. It doesn't want to admit that practitioners don't know enough about RSIs to treat them or that these injuries don't generate enough profit to justify figuring out how. At the same time, the establishment doesn't want to cede territory to holistic medicine either, so it fights patients on the one hand and the insurance industry on the other. Doctors fight with doctors. Practitioners discredit each other. Patients battle doctors and insurance companies. Unions lock horns with big business. By the time government steps in, you have a full-blown political circus controlled by high-dollar special interests.

To my mind, this really comes down to an enormous financial interest in there being no scientific evidence that work causes stress, which causes injury. The colloquial term for RSIs contains two of those words. Some systems in other countries have gone so far as to change the terminology and methods of reporting to hide the implications. England, for example, does not cover RSIs under its national health-care system, so any sufferer must go outside the system to seek treatment or get no care at all. If able to draw a definitive connection between musculoskeletal pain and stress on the job, medical science would establish a legal basis for concluding that stress at work causes occupational illness. Imagine the claims that would follow. Would we then try to limit the amount of work we may do? Would we be forced to cap our productivity just as other countries are surpassing us with theirs? Wouldn't that affect our gross national product? Our entire economy is built on the idea of limitless expansion.

The evidence is already there, but no one's collecting it in such a way that those conclusions can be drawn. So, RSIs have remained the number one occupational illness in the country for over twenty years largely because the insurance-pharmaceutical-political complex is doing everything possible not to solve the problem. Meanwhile, millions of dollars and productive lives are being wasted. Powerful interests face off against the little guy, although the sides the players are on might surprise you.

The Occupational Safety and Health Administration (OSHA) has tried to tackle RSIs through public policy for thirty years in a tale worthy of a Dickens novel. Labor first approached OSHA about RSIs in the early 1980s when incidents had increased 1,000 percent.[1] OSHA opened joint discussions with unions and big business. Lawmakers backed by big business dug in deep, contending that there was no scientific evidence showing that jobs involving repetitive motion cause musculoskeletal disorders. The opposition, comprising lawmakers backed by unions, was equally entrenched. The National Academy of Sciences decided to conduct what was supposed to be a definitive study. Finally, in 1999, almost twenty years later, the Clinton administration was coming to an end, and everyone was rushing to get their paperwork finished before the new president took office.

As OSHA is an administration, its rulings do not need to be passed by legislation. To block OSHA's attempts to mitigate the incidence of work-related RSIs, Congress tried to enact a law prohibiting the use of federal funds to propose or enforce any ergonomics standard, effectively defunding any standard OSHA might intend to publish. But the National Academy of Sciences couldn't complete its study in time, and Congress adjourned before completing its bill, so Secretary of Labor Alexis Herman published OSHA's ergonomic standards in January 2000, making them law.[2]

Four days after George W. Bush became president, the newly convened Republican Congress invoked the never-before-used Congressional Review Act to overturn the ergonomic standards. The Republican Congress went even further, making it illegal for OSHA to propose any rule substantially similar to the former one; the administration has been effectively hog-tied ever since. By this time, the National Academy of Sciences' had released its study concluding that there were simply too many other factors to blame musculoskeletal pain merely on a repetitive-motion job. The definitive study was inconclusive; yet the National Academy of Sciences never performed another.

THE AUSTRALIA PHENOMENON

At the same time, similar forces were converging in countries all over the world, with varying success. But nowhere did the drama become as Dickensian as it did in Australia, which experienced a sudden spike in musculoskeletal pain among keyboard operators at Australia Telecomm between 1984 and 1985. In 1987, just as suddenly, these claims stopped. Officials blamed the doctors, the unions, the media, and "occupational hysteria" because nearly all the sufferers were female. They attacked RSIs on three fronts, stating that the injuries did not exist; or if they did exist, they were stress-related mental conditions; and any physical injuries were really due to activities the injured worker performed away from the job, like gardening. In response, the Australian workers' compensation system changed its definition of what constituted a compensable injury and stopped covering RSIs in 1987.[3] But did that get rid of the problem?

The brave folks at the RSI and Overuse Injury Association of the Australian Capital Territories, the only surviving RSI support group in the country, has kept tabs on the problem, continuing to provide help to sufferers there. The tracking of RSIs in Australia now varies from territory to territory. They are sometimes called musculoskeletal disorders (MSDs) or occupational overuse syndrome; sometimes they fall under the rubric of "body stressing," a term the workers' compensation system in Australia uses to obscure RSIs. It defines body stressing as derived from occupations that require "manual handling, repetitive movement, and/or the maintenance of constrained or awkward postures."[4] In 2012, 80 percent of public servants in the Australian Capital Territory suffered from occupational overuse syndrome; 87.2 percent of dentists in Queensland experienced an MSD; of Australia's eight full-time professional orchestras, 84 percent of members experienced pain or injuries that interfered with their work; and 95 percent of sonographers suffered from an MSD.[5] Body stressing accounted for 43 percent of all serious injury claims in 2010 and 2011.[6] The total cost for body-stressing injuries and illnesses countrywide in 2008 and 2009 was AU$25.2 million.[7] Changing the definition, clearly does not make RSIs go away.

Here in the United States, Arkansas has tried a similar tactic. Its workers' compensation system limits coverage of RSIs to repetitive motion for back or neck and hearing. Texas allows companies to opt out of the workers' compensation system altogether. But unlike in other states that permit self-insurers, in Texas companies can actually change what injuries are compensable, as well as how much compensation a worker can receive. This means they can refuse to provide lifetime coverage and can force arbitration,[8] whereby employers make a "take-it-or-leave-it" offer and the injured worker has no recourse in the state system. To make matters worse, in 1989 Texas essentially barred its attorneys from practicing in the workers' compensation arena, "frequently resulting in the worker being denied justice without any practical recourse."[9] Ironically, in 2005, the Texas legislature finally acknowledged the need to provide injured workers with legal help.[10] Disturbingly, the state of Oklahoma in 2013 adopted Texas's opt-out program in what the insurance industry hopes will be a wave that sweeps the nation.

WHAT WAS WRONG WITH OSHA'S ERGONOMICS STANDARDS

OSHA's ergonomics standards were far from perfect. They required employers to make up the difference between injured workers' regular pay and their earnings from the lower-paying jobs they were forced to take, as well as to supplement injured workers' regular salaries if they became permanently disabled due to an RSI. Both requirements were unprecedented and should fall within the domain of workers' compensation insurance; employers would be double dipped, paying for insurance premiums that are supposed to cover the injury and then paying the injured worker as well. Big business decried the cost, with estimates reaching $4.5 billion annually, though many industries expected them to be much higher.

The ergonomic standards set up a complicated reporting system but would not have educated the public or prevented the injuries. In fact, they wouldn't even kick in until a second worker got an RSI in the same company. OSHA usually holds employers responsible for identifying and correcting hazards before an injury occurs, not after. OSHA continues to enforce ergonomic standards via its general duties rule, under which employers have "an obligation to keep the workplace free from recognized serious hazards, including ergonomic hazards."[11] In 2010, OSHA came at the problem from a new direction by changing how RSIs are reported. Whereas they used to be lumped under "general injury" or "other," they now have their own category. This will entail lots more paperwork, but it also means more data can be collected about RSIs in the workplace. Trying to access even more data, OSHA has most recently proposed requiring large companies to make their injury records public.[12]

WHO'S CONTROLLING THE DATA

I'm no scientist, but if the National Academy of Sciences study didn't reveal whether work predominantly causes RSIs or hobbies such as guitar picking, video editing, and woodworking contribute to them, then it would make sense to do another study. It hasn't. It seems pretty obvious to me that if you're typing forty hours a week and gardening for two, gardening isn't the source of the problem. Also, you can always stop gardening, but you can't stop working. On the other hand, if you're texting the boss ten times a day, then playing drums for a heavy metal band on the weekends, your day job isn't causing the injury either. I'm certain a roomful of lawyers could come up with a schedule for this. Other factors, such as age and weight, also seem to play a role and present an even stickier problem. Which came first, the obesity or the sedentary job? If your only meal options during your fifteen-minute lunch come out of a vending machine in the break room, who's responsible for your food choices, you or your employer?

Double-blind studies are expensive and take a long time to conduct. Because studies cost so much money, only institutions with deep pockets, like insurance and pharmaceutical companies and universities, can afford to conduct them. They're the ones who establish the hypotheses for examination and thereby even control what data becomes available. There are lots of RSI studies, for instance, on carpal tunnel release surgery versus wrist bracing but none on carpal tunnel release surgery versus acupuncture. The acupuncturists aren't organized or rich enough to fund such a study, and the resulting data could be counterproductive to the surgeons who could afford to fund it.

Small studies compare yoga to wrist bracing, acupuncture to steroid injections, and Active Release Techniques to no treatment at all, but small studies only provide enough data to suggest that further studies are warranted. Instead, we need comprehensive studies comparing the different RSIs, habits of patients, and various treatments. Thus far, this has meant that the availability of data is controlled by those who have a strong financial incentive not to produce it. The result is a phrase that drives me crazy: there's no medical evidence to support that.

When Arnold Schwarzenegger decided to reform the California workers' compensation system, one area he wanted to address was chiropractic. A study had revealed that injured workers received significantly more chiropractic treatments in California than in other states.[13] So he limited the number of visits to the chiropractor per patient to twenty-four.[14] His decision did not take into account, however, how much money those visits to the chiropractor actually saved versus surgery. That's because the chiropractors in California didn't spend enough on lobbyists at the time.

You know who else doesn't spend as much money on lobbyists as doctors, hospitals, and pharmaceutical and insurance companies? Everyone else in the health-care system. It seems to me that, with the backing of so many deep pockets, if studies had shown that RSIs are significantly attributable to hobbies rather than work, this data would be available. Many insurance companies will only say that "a definite causal link between computer use and musculoskeletal injuries has eluded scientists."[15]

CROWD SOURCING MEDICAL STUDIES

We can also harness the very technology that caused RSI sufferers their injuries in the first place to solve this problem effectively through crowd sourcing and open sourcing. Jay Bradner, a researcher at Harvard and Dana Farber in Boston, gave a talk at TedX in 2011 about how he and his team were able to use open sourcing to develop a new cancer drug. Once they had developed a prototype, instead of keeping it a secret and patenting it, as pharmaceutical companies do, they actually published a paper, including the chemical composition of their prototype, and told people how to make it. Forty labs in the United States and thirty more in Europe began studying the prototype, developing a whole bunch of new applications that the original lab might not have discovered on its own. The results yielded a much quicker, much cheaper business model for discovering a new drug. Along the way, these researchers discovered something far more valuable than the drug alone: a new resource for drug discovery. Bradner says, "If anything is unique about this research, it's less the science than the strategy—that this for us was a social experiment."[16]

Crowd sourcing, another tool whereby data is collected from a large number of people, is being used at AOMA Graduate School of Integrative Medicine in Austin, Texas. AOMA treats twenty thousand patients annually on its two campuses, providing acupuncture, herbology, nutritional counseling, and other Eastern medical therapies. It has integrated software into its records system to collect data from patients who opt into the program. This data is part of the usual exam routine anyway; AOMA is just digitizing it. Imagine if it partnered with every other acupuncture school in the United States? Imagine if a group of RSI practitioners did the same thing. Imagine how easy it would be to add variables into such a system that its original design omitted, such as the types of leisure activities patients enjoy on weekends.

"Gathering information from ordinary citizens across the world has the potential to accelerate the pace of health-care research of all kinds," says a team from the Perelman School of Medicine at the University of Pennsylvania. "It could even improve the quality of research while reducing the costs."[17] Yet, the Penn team cautions that the technique is new, and little is known about its potential. The team calls for standardized guidelines to ensure a consistent quality of data.

The State Pain Policy Advocacy Network (SPPAN) is using open sourcing in a low-tech way. SPPAN saw a need for collaboration and coordination of pain policy at the state level. Organizations often don't have the staff to do what they want locally. The information necessary to make these organizations effective is fragmented and inconsistent. Sound familiar? Organizations like SPPAN work to bridge the gap, creating a much stronger force. Other organizations with similar interests could take a page from SPPAN's playbook. As for how this might help RSI sufferers, Director Amy Goldstein says, "We're seeing more workers' compensation issues coming through legislatures."[18]

SMALL BUSINESS SUFFERS AS MUCH AS PATIENTS

The patsy in all this is not just injured workers; it's also employers. President George W. Bush's labor secretary, Elaine Chao, did set public hearings in the summer of 2001 to "look into the matter" of ergonomics. I attended the California forum to see for myself why everyone is fighting so hard against having any standards. After enumerating all the efforts by OSHA to counter the problem, one panelist quipped, "What else do we need to do, put up billboards?" Dr. Peter Mandel, from the American Academy of Orthopedic Surgeons, heartily replied, "Yes!"[19]

The conference made clear that small businesses are left in the lurch. Large corporations have a much greater chance of seeing these injuries and their destructive consequences. But small employers with only one or two workers in dangerous jobs find out about RSIs the hard way—after an employee develops one. These injuries can bankrupt a small company. Powerful lobbies, like the US Chamber of Commerce, have pressed hard to exempt small enterprises from any ergonomics standards; yet they have done their constituents a disservice by failing to arm them with vital information that could literally save their companies, as well as their employees.

Small businesses make up 99.7 percent of employers in the United States.[20] What's worse, over three-quarters of small businesses are basically one-man shops. So, what if you are the one employee in your company to get an RSI? What if, to cut costs, you were forced to opt out of any workers' compensation insurance? What if you don't have any health insurance at all?

The sheer logistics of reaching millions of people has kept OSHA's focus on large corporations and union employees. Consequently, most white-collar workers, who are particularly susceptible to RSIs, have been left completely out of the picture. As a Los Angeles RSI Support Group white paper pointed out, "Everyone wants the same thing: as few injuries as possible, for as little cost as possible, with the quickest returns to work as possible."[21]

All this may seem like a perfect storm, but the perfect storm has only begun to gather. What will happen when the next generation, weaned on technology, enters the workforce?

Part 3

THE SOCIAL IMPACT OF RSIs

Chapter Nine

Teens and Texting

Repetitive strain injuries have been around since the earliest days of recorded history. They become problematic whenever there's a major advancement in society, then fade away once the latest invention is replaced with a better one, such as the telephone replacing the telegraph. Children are often exploited during these advancements until society steps in to protect its future. In the instance of our current technological revolution, however, we're seeing a particularly unusual phenomenon as one advancement, the information age, begets a second, the knowledge age—a double evolution, if you will. This time, instead of just one, we're about to see two and possibly three generations falling prey to RSIs if we don't address the problem.

We find the earliest evidence of a repetitive task causing pain in ancient Egypt, where court scribes routinely fell prey to the hand cramps of what we now call focal dystonia. RSIs first appeared in world medical literature in the seventeenth century when milkmaids reported the arm and wrist pain of what we have been calling tendonitis. During the Industrial Revolution, the RSI of the day was telegrapher's wrist, or what we now call carpal tunnel syndrome. RSIs have steadily remained the bane of the shop floor ever since. All that has changed is who's getting RSIs and how many people are getting them.

Once personal computers became a mainstay of the workplace, RSIs began to skyrocket; by 1994 they had increased 1,000 percent.[1] Because white-collar clerical workers and women, who make up less than half of the workforce but suffered two-thirds of all ergonomic injuries in 2002, were mostly affected, it was easy to blame the epidemic on hysteria. Once the Internet became a pervasive tool in the workplace, members of white-collar occupations considered far removed from manual labor began to develop RSIs, and a second wave attacked high-paying technical and executive workers. A third wave is just beginning as tablets allow us to go paperless. The deliveryman, utility worker, and Apple Store employee all use tablets now as part of their jobs. Indeed, does any job today not require the regular, repeated use of some type of technology?

In the past, RSIs faded once technology advanced enough (e.g., with the advent of mechanical milking equipment, dairymaids developed less tendonitis). During the current revolution, however, new inventions rely increasingly on hand operation and are less ergonomically sound; worse, they have fostered an insidious addiction as we all become technology dependent. Nowhere is this addiction more prevalent than in the fourth wave of injuries that's about to hit our children.

TEENS AND TEXTING

In its landmark 2010 study, "Media in the Lives of 8 to 18 Year Olds," the Kaiser Family Foundation found that children spend an average of two hours, forty-two minutes with their computers and video games in a typical day.[2] They also found children spend an average of two hours, eleven minutes a day talking, listening to music, watching TV and videos, and playing games on their cell phones.[3] This number does not take into account the hour and a half per day that twelve- to eighteen-year-olds spend texting.[4] That adds up to six hours, twenty-three minutes a day using technology. By way of comparison, Liberty Mutual's comprehensive study on ergonomics and computer use in the workplace defined a heavy user as one who spends more than four hours a day at the computer.[5] By the time your twelve-year-old enters the workforce, he will have already been a heavy computer user for six to ten years.

Lest you think the computer keyboard is the only culprit, Jeff Teideman, loss-control consultant at California's State Compensation Insurance Fund, points out that we hold our smart phones in a static position, gripping it, potentially for long periods. Even if we perform the activity off and on, at six hours, twenty-three minutes a day, "I think you're going to start seeing a lot more prevalence of problems as a result of this," says Teideman.[6]

Studies into the effects of technology on teens are in their infancy, but there are already terms for the RSIs kids are developing: texting tendonitis, text neck, and texting thumb. At current count, only around ten papers report a correlation between texting and tendonitis, with most sufferers being under twenty-one.[7] Judith Gold, the author of one such study, is a software engineer turned occupational epidemiologist and ergonomist. The similarities between people using computers and people using handheld devices seemed apparent to her. Both use their fingers to type on some sort of keyboard, and both hold their shoulders and neck in a static position.

In her small study, Gold found that people who texted more per day were at greater risk for neck and shoulder pain. Her study represents the barest beginning of a scientific correlation. A study in Ontario correlated the number of text messages and duration of texting with pain in the base of the thumb.[8] Gold speaks emphatically: "We do not yet understand the causes. This is a nascent area of research."[9] Gold points out that very few studies on computer use have looked at college students as well as adults. How do we know what the outcome of all this early technology use will be?

In the absence of research, we can only extrapolate to get an idea of what kind of problem we could be facing when our tech-savvy teens enter the workforce. A person operating a handheld device for six hours, twenty-three minutes per day spends 50 percent more time using technology than the average heavy computer user at work today. According to the American College of Rheumatology, 4 to 10 million Americans suffer from carpal tunnel syndrome and other RSIs,[10] and according to Nolo's legal encyclopedia, one in eight American workers are affected.[11] A 50 percent increase in those numbers would mean 6 to 15 million Americans, or one in six workers, were affected. RSIs would represent 90 percent of all work-related injuries, and create more than 35 million new permanently disabled Americans.[12] Will we be creating a disabled workforce under the age of twenty-five?

BONNIE'S STORY

Bonnie Prestridge is a twenty-five-year-old worker disabled by RSIs. She got them when she was eighteen through a combination of schoolwork and piano playing. She underwent various treatments, including movement retraining, and adapted as best she could, but she continued to experience reinjuries. While studying at the University of California, Berkeley, Bonnie developed a second type of RSI that we have not yet talked about: vocal chord strain from using voice-recognition software. Bonnie had to leave school midway through her sophomore year and return to her parents' home to heal.

"I was like an infant," says Bonnie. "I relied on my parents to wash my hair, to feed me."[13] Bonnie's parents were very supportive, and her doctors were considered very good, but her insurance did not cover the therapies that helped. None of her practitioners could crack her RSIs. After eighteen months, Bonnie returned to college, but then she had to leave again for a semester when her voice again became disabled, before she finally finished her degree at Berkeley.

After six years, Bonnie lost all hope of ever being able to hold a job or lead the life she had envisioned. She finally found an internship in Washington, DC, with the Department of Labor's Office of Disability Employment Policy, where her experiences were valued. Bonnie, a self-ascribed type A personality, says that, prior to her injury, she derived her sense of self from achieving. Then she had to drop all the activities that brought her fulfillment—piano, which she had studied since age four, school, sports, painting. Keeping motivated throughout her injury was particularly difficult. "Disability isn't just physical, it's also social," says Bonnie.[14] When asked about the future of RSIs given all the teen texting, Bonnie says, "It's like this time bomb just waiting to go off."[15]

The youngest subject of the Ontario teens-and-texting study was fourteen years old. There has also been a report of a thirteen year old from Dallas getting texting tendonitis.[16] The youngest member of the Los Angeles RSI Support Group was twelve. Her story is a lot like Bonnie's: she spent two to three hours a day doing homework on the computer and another several hours practicing the cello. Her disability just began six years sooner. Movement-retraining specialist Greg Dempster's youngest client is an eight-year-old video game enthusiast. When he developed tendonitis, his parents made him reduce his game time and called on Dempster to retrain him. "We came up with a solution for using his gaming console so he could play without injury," says Dempster, "but he hated it because it slowed him down."[17]

When such teens enter the workforce, their injuries will be considered preexisting conditions. The workers' compensation system is not included under the Affordable Care Act. Because RSIs are cumulative traumas, occurring over time and not always attributable to work, chances are that future injured workers will have even greater difficulty receiving treatment through the workers' compensation system. Indeed, Jeff Teideman at California's State Compensation Insurance Fund sees a frightening situation ahead. "By the time eighteen- to nineteen-year-olds hit the job market, they may already be injured or well on their way to an injury. I don't know where that's going to go."[18] If the injuries are even somewhat attributable to work, their regular health insurance will not cover them either. They could get caught in a battle between insurance companies, and we've already seen what delays in treatment do to RSIs.

The good news is that, as of 2008, when your injured teen enters the workforce as a disabled employee, the Americans with Disabilities Act (ADA) will cover those RSI sufferers whose disability affects all their life activities, not just job-related ones. The bad news is that unemployment rates for the disabled remain as high as 70 percent for individuals with severe disabilities.[19] Another statistic to consider is that the ADA applies only to businesses with fifteen employees or more, and small businesses provide 67 percent of all first jobs,[20] so your texting teen may never even get into the workforce.

HOW DO YOU STOP THEM?

I posed this question to everyone I interviewed, and the response was a resounding "Gee, that's a tough one." Dempster admits that his video game enthusiast would not have agreed to adjust his play if his parents hadn't sat on him. Ergonomist and epidemiologist Judith Gold says children present a particular problem when it comes to prevention because they think they're invincible. "I can't get adults to understand this. How do you get a child to understand it?" says Gold.[21] Is this really a choice between work and play? Can we tell an entire generation of kids they have to choose between the two?

There's a way to play the piano so that the activity won't hurt you. There is also a way to use a standard computer keyboard without getting injured. But the design of gaming consoles doesn't allow for healthy play. Nor are smart phones designed for use without causing injury. And the jury is still out on tablets. Education—such as informing users to get off the mouse as much as possible—would certainly help. Bonnie's story illustrates the limits of voice-recognition software as an alternative to keying. Parents can attempt to limit their child's access to these technologies, to cap the number of hours they play them, and to insist that their children vary their activities. But something else is operating here beyond the need for parental involvement, education, and better industrial design.

Digital devices have become an unprecedentedly ubiquitous and integral part of our world. We can only compare them to television; yet television was an entertainment device, not also a requisite social, communications, and work tool. The similarity lies in their addictiveness. The most common elements of addiction shed some light on why teens are particularly susceptible: feelings of pleasure or changes in mood, psychological dependence, changes in the brain, and painful withdrawal.

The brain is attracted to movement. It has to process what it sees, which is why you can't take your eyes off the television. Between fast, MTV-inspired edits, text constantly running along the bottom of the screen, and pop-ups, today's television involves significantly more movement than it did even five years ago. Yet TV viewing is still passive, whereas the new technologies are all about viewer participation and gamification (e.g., "click to learn more," "buy now," and so forth). It seems that this added dimension will make our devices even more addicting than television. We all know adults who can't separate themselves from their BlackBerries, but with teens you get another component. Humans begin the process of individuation during their teens. Teenagers now build their sense of self through social media—they display whom and what they know and what they like publicly through everything they do on their devices. They are absolutely psychologically dependent on them. The ongoing conversation acts like a serial soap opera. Their minds are never fully able to process all the information because it's always being updated.

All this interacting is also changing their brains. So much information is contained in one screen, with each bit stimulating the brain and requiring processing. Anything less information dense is boring to young people who have grown up with this technology. This level of interaction with devices is also changing the delicate chemical balance in our bodies as the stimulus triggers oversecretion of certain neurotransmitters and hormones, throwing our whole bodies out of whack and making us need more stimulation to maintain homeostasis. This is also one of the components of addiction.

Stopping your child's addiction then would require that you change her psychological dependence and teach her how to develop a sense of self outside technology. This, of course, would require that you also derive your sense of self outside technology. As for the brain changes, stopping your child's addiction would require returning her brain chemistry to the optimal homeostasis. Paul Graham, in his compelling essay "The Acceleration of Addictiveness," says he's switched from running to taking long hikes because the slowness allows him to think more. Find things your children like to do that are slow and removed from technology. Graham believes that in an age of accelerated everything, "we'll increasingly be defined by what we say no to."[22]

What is a good way to stop your and your teen's addiction to technology? Just as with RSIs, I'm afraid, there is no magic pill. Appendix B contains a number of tools for parents to start educating their children and to begin the conversation within the family.

The Industrial Revolution rode in on the backs of children. By 1910, 2 million children under the age of fifteen were employed in factories in the United States.[23] In a similar way, teens are pivotal to today's development of new media as an enterprise—this time not as workers but as consumers. Children spend $4.2 billion per year of their own money consuming.[24] They also influence their parents' purchases. A 2012 study by Nickelodeon finds that parents solicit their children's opinions in 49 percent of mobile phone purchases. When it comes to all other purchases, that number jumps to 95 percent.[25]

The Nickelodeon study holds a clue about how to slow children's technology usage. Parents and children in the new millennium have a very different sort of relationship than in past generations. Today the majority of decision making within families involves the children's input.[26] If you consider everything presented in this book, you'll realize that RSIs are a family affair, and you'll call a family meeting.

Chapter Ten

Employers and RSIs

Ultimately, repetitive strain injuries also leave employers holding the bag. Worker safety standards protect them as well. But until an employee files a claim, most companies don't measure the costs of an injured employee. The Occupational Safety and Health Administration (OSHA) brought ergonomics programs to nearly half a million workers; yet sheer logistics forced the administration to limit its programs to employees of large corporations and union members. Consequently, most white-collar workers and small businesses, which are particularly vulnerable to RSI, have been left completely out of the picture.

Instead of pointing fingers at each other, workers and businesses should team up. That's the only way the problem will get solved. Larger companies already know this and are taking matters into their own hands. Chapter 5 on ergonomics makes clear that workers share some responsibility in this situation. Now, let's turn to what employers can do—because there is a lot.

A CLOG IN THE INFORMATION PIPELINE

OSHA does a great job working with big companies and in industry sectors. Its most recent ergonomics program targets the health-care industry, where musculoskeletal disorders account for as many as 20 percent of nurses' injuries; the cost of back injuries alone is estimated at $20 billion annually.[1] It is attacking the problem in five states, working closely with unions, employers, and professional associations. OSHA has a fine history of working with groups to solve occupational safety problems. It falls short, however, when it comes to smaller businesses, particularly those without any union employees or professional associations. Unfortunately, this is where the first wave of

RSIs hit the hardest. Small businesses represent 99.7 percent of all employers in the United States and more than 50 percent of the private workforce. [2]

There are two reasons for this: logistics and a bill that the Republicans pushed through Congress in their successful quashing of OSHA's ergonomics standards back in 2000. That bill made it illegal for the government to fund enforcement of any ergonomics program. OSHA simply doesn't have the money to get the word out about prevention. By targeting large companies, unions, and professional associations, the administration does a remarkable job of reaching as many workers as it does.

The US Chamber of Commerce, a major lobby group that supported that bill, joined congressional Republicans in their historical effort to stop the ergonomic standards, all in the name of saving small businesses. Unfortunately, the Chamber hung their own constituents out to dry in the process and continue to do so to this day by failing to provide adequate ergonomic information and assistance to the 25 million small businesses in the United States.

If you go to its website, you'll find that the US Chamber of Commerce continues to fight costly lawsuits on behalf of small businesses. An article at the Friends of the US Chamber of Commerce states that more than two-thirds of small business owners say they would have to "hold back on hiring new employees, cut benefits and raise costs for consumers if targeted by a lawsuit."[3] Let me be very clear here: any workers' compensation claim for an RSI is a lawsuit. These pages demonstrate the likelihood that a small business will become the target of one of these lawsuits. What greater threat to small businesses exists? To my mind, the US Chamber of Commerce has seriously dropped the ball.

Workers' compensation insurance companies are also supposed to provide loss-prevention information to their policyholders. In California, it's against the law for them not to do so. Most larger workers' compensation carriers have conducted their own in-house research on ergonomics and published materials on their results. Many workers' compensation insurance companies across the nation offer occupational health and safety services and will send a specialist to audit your workplace to assist you in developing an ergonomics program for your company.

This is what Jeff Teideman does for California's State Compensation Insurance Fund, but he includes a caveat: "We've known for years that when we do ergonomics training for employers, there will be a spike in RSI claims for that company." Companies are afraid of that spike, but as Teideman sees it, the claims would have been made anyway. Statistics show that costs are significantly lower once an employer sets up earlier interventions. "In the end, it's way more cost-effective, even though there's a spike," says Teideman. [4]

Teideman encourages companies to develop an in-house program they can run themselves. He helps them set up an ergonomics task force, generally comprising four to six people whom he trains in detail; they then become the ergonomics experts for the company. He says it's a great way to raise awareness, as well as a good team-building exercise for the workers. He also finds that this approach keeps the spikes down.

All of these services are free, but you probably are not aware of them. That's because, once again, logistics make it far easier to approach large companies, unions, and professional associations when providing the information and training necessary to educate employers. Teidcman occasionally provides workshops on ergonomics for small businesses, but there is not much demand, and his territory spans half the state. You can contact your workers' compensation carrier or your state's workers' compensation office for more information. If more small businesses request the services, I'm sure carriers will be only too happy to provide them. Doing so reduces their costs too.

GETTING BETTER OUTCOMES FROM THE WORKERS' COMPENSATION SYSTEM

Employers are paying for a workers' compensation system that fails to provide acceptable return-to-work outcomes. Yet, when it comes to claims management, they are the most silent. The numbers should make clear that current outcomes are unacceptable. This is owing largely, in my view, to claims management, where the singular goal of reducing claims costs has clouded the larger picture.

Employers can do a lot to help. When a carrier investigates an employee's injury, rather than denying it in the heat of the moment, conduct a little investigation of your own. Such an investigation would include educating yourself about RSIs, as well as evaluating that employee's workstation, workload, and work process. Once a claim has been filed, employers can request that their insurance carrier keep them apprised of how it is progressing so that an equitable solution can be achieved.

Insurance carriers have a duty to act in good faith on behalf of the policyholder, the employer. Although an injured worker cannot hold a workers' compensation insurance carrier to the good faith requirement, an employer can. Employer intervention would go a long way toward improving return-to-work outcomes for RSIs. Once your employee is medically cleared to return to work, your part in the process becomes crucial. Everyone I talk to on the RSI front lines cites employer cooperation as crucial to successful return-to-work outcomes. That means having patience, often redesigning the work process, and sometimes even redesigning the boss. Human beings do not generally like change, but if we are going to tackle this problem, change is necessary. When we get to the work-redesign section in chapter 12, we'll see how this can increase a company's productivity, profitability, and valuation.

WHAT YOU CAN DO TO PREVENT RSIS

Large employers who are also self-insured have seen the positive results of cooperating with RSI-injured workers. Their claims managers understand what getting everyone back up to full speed will take. In fact, they are so aware of how much RSIs will cost them that they invest substantially in prevention.

Another prevention tool entails addressing a gap in care in the current workers' compensation system: the point between an employee's feeling pain and having to file a workers' compensation claim. Midsize companies are able to fill this gap in care by hiring an occupational nurse and having an on-site clinic. Not every company can afford an on-site clinic, however, so Dr. P. Michael Leahy took his Active Release Techniques (ART) to industrial settings as first aid. Beginning in 2002, OSHA exempted injuries requiring only first aid from reporting. So long as no time away from work or medical care, among other things, is required, injuries are considered treatable with first aid. Practitioners licensed in ART can provide on-site massages on a scheduled basis, or they can provide first aid services to businesses near their offices so that employees can get a massage during their lunch hour or before or after work.[5] These first aid treatments are at the employer's expense but oftentimes can be covered under the company health-care policy. When ART intervention is applied during the first aid stage, discomfort can be resolved after four to six treatments of about fifteen minutes each.[6] "That's a proactive safety program," says ergonomist and movement-retraining specialist Greg Dempster.[7] The program is so successful that ART is an OSHA-approved treatment and considered a management best practice.

DEVELOPING AN ERGONOMICS PROGRAM
FOR SMALL BUSINESS

Small businesses without the financial wherewithal to adopt any of these safety measures can still develop an inexpensive in-house prevention program that works. Small businesses enjoy a number of advantages in this regard. They are far more nimble; they can respond much more quickly and harness the closer relationships they have with their employees. Small employers often know their workers' families—whose spouse is sick and whose kid is applying to college. This makes the team approach to RSI prevention so much more powerful than in a larger company.

Foremost in such a program, then, is the idea that employees are assets, not liabilities. If you treat your employees like liabilities, that's what they will be; if you treat them as assets, they will be assets. Your employees are the cheapest way of developing an RSI-prevention program because you harness their brainpower, experience, and perspective, all key to creative problem solving. Ergonomist and epidemiologist Judith Gold uses the participatory ergonomics approach. "It's really the people who are doing the job that know best how to perform that job," she says.[8] The workers who actually have the aches and pains also probably have some idea of what's causing them. Gold taps them for ideas about how to improve working conditions.

As an additional benefit, the participatory ergonomics approach actually reduces the amount of stress your employees experience in the workplace. Studies have shown that job stress comes not only from the demands placed on the employee but also from the amount of control a worker has over how to perform assigned tasks.[9] Furthermore, studies by the National Institute of Occupational Safety and Health show that job stress increases the risk of RSIs.[10] So giving your employees greater control over how they perform their work will actually reduce their stress and susceptibility to injury. The Centers for Disease Control website provides a step-by-step guide to preventing job stress, along with example solutions other small businesses have developed. More information is also provided in appendix C.

Another benefit of implementing an ergonomics program at your business is that OSHA sees doing so as a good faith effort to abate hazards, and it'll save you a citation should one of your employees develop an RSI.

WHAT MAKES A GOOD ERGONOMIC INTERVENTION PROGRAM

Liberty Mutual Insurance Company, the largest workers' compensation carrier in the country, is one of the few with its own research department. In 2000 it studied what makes an effective ergonomic intervention program. "Simply providing adjustable furniture is not effective," says Dr. Marvin Dainoff, PhD, director of the Research Institute's Center for Behavioral Sciences, Liberty Mutual's research arm.[11] Employers must also understand the context within which their ergonomic interventions are to be implemented. This means considering the people, technology, work processes, and management structures necessary to achieve a healthy workplace. The study compared three different types of interventions: adjustable workstations, training, and no intervention at all. The ergonomic intervention that saw greatest improvement of symptoms was adjustable workstations combined with training.

It's important to note that many of these solutions are low-cost, often requiring nothing more than a few meetings, open lines of communication, and creativity.

Chapter Eleven

Why RSIs Cost You, Even if You Don't Have One

According to the Occupational Safety and Health Administration (OSHA), repetitive strain injuries cost the United States approximately $20 billion per year in workers' compensation expenditures.[1] A 2008 Microsoft study says RSIs cost businesses over $600 million in lost work hours.[2] The National Academy of Sciences says RSIs drain approximately $50 billion from the American economy annually.[3] As staggering as these numbers are, they do not include many of the hidden costs of RSIs. Whether or not you, a loved one, or an employee has contracted an RSI, whether or not you even believe in RSIs, they are still costing you. And if a number of current trends continue unabated, RSIs are about to cost us a whole lot more.

COST SHIFTING THE DISABLED FROM WORKERS' COMPENSATION TO SOCIAL SECURITY

Chief among these trends is cost shifting. Reforms in the state-run workers' compensation systems in the last twenty years have come from insurance industry–backed measures that reduce costs by "shifting them to other publically funded programs like Social Security and Medicare,"[4] says Cathy Stanton of the Workers Injury Law and Advocacy Group. Once state-run workers' compensation programs began utilizing only American Medical Association–established treatment guidelines and capping permanent disability payments and future medical care, the workers' compensation system covered fewer and fewer workers' injuries and forced more and more injured workers onto Social Security Disability Insurance (SSDI). One report says that occupational injuries and illnesses result in costs well over three times the amounts published. [5]

RSIs have to comprise a significant portion of this cost shifting, as they represent 60 percent of occupational injuries, are often disallowed or undertreated by the workers' compensation system, and are three times more likely to result in a permanent disability than any other occupational injury or illness. In the journal *New Solutions: A Journal of Environmental and Occupational Health Policy*, Joseph LaDou of the University of California, San Francisco, School of Medicine writes, "Most of the responsibility for compensating disabled workers now resides in the federal government, not in the state systems." [6]

An article in the *Journal of Occupational and Environmental Medicine* goes further, stating that most occupational injuries and illnesses aren't covered by the workers' compensation system at all anymore. [7] Most disabled workers go to Social Security and Medicare, but an estimated 2 million more have to rely on something else for their health care, with costs exceeding $11 billion. [8]

So it is not surprising that a record one in fourteen workers now participates in the SSDI program. [9] During the period from January 2009 through September 2013, 5.9 million new people were added to the SSDI roles. [10] News reports blame all the recently unemployed workers who can't find a job. These publications, however, fail to do their research. One cannot simply go from being employed to unemployed to disabled. A rigorous, two-year process to qualify for SSDI requires input from doctors, lawyers, and employment experts, as well as a high standard of proof, all of which someone who's been in the workers' compensation system already has. An article at Catholic Online goes so far as to say, "Somebody is fleecing the system, or at least trying very hard to do so." [11] That somebody is the states' workers' compensation systems.

How much of this can be blamed on RSIs? Over the past thirty years, the number of persons disabled due to musculoskeletal disorders increased from 13 to 28 percent. [12] In another report, 33.8 percent of newly diagnosed disabled workers suffered from back pain and other musculoskeletal problems in 2011. [13] Although the injuries these numbers represent are not necessarily all attributable to RSIs, and although experts have not directly calculated how much the swell in the SSDI rolls stems from cost shifting by the nation's workers' compensation system, according to LaDou, SSDI now pays four times more in disability costs than all the states' workers' compensation programs combined. [14]

Injured workers denied care by the workers' compensation system are entitled to Medicare as well as SSDI benefits. Medicare is largely set up for senior populations. The only RSI treatments covered are surgery, physical therapy, and, in some cases, chiropractic. So RSI sufferers kicked onto SSDI have virtually no opportunity to recover. It is no wonder then that SSDI returns only 6 percent of its patients to work, and only 3.6 percent improve enough from the medical care they receive on Medicare that they are no longer disabled.[15]

SSDI is funded by a 1.8 percent payroll tax on you, costing taxpayers $128.9 billion in 2011. If you are an employer, you pay twice, for both workers' compensation insurance and SSDI. If you are an employer who develops an RSI, you pay four times because the injured worker has to pay Medicare in order to receive any health-care benefits, and Medicare also seeks redress from the employers for all this cost shifting. Social Security got wind of the fast one the workers' compensation insurers were pulling and started requiring that injured workers pay Medicare part of their workers' compensation settlement to cover future health-care costs, even though Medicare does not adequately cover RSI care. That portion is sometimes as great as 75 percent of the injured worker's award! Medicare can further require reimbursement for all workers' compensation–related medical care payments from the employer who oversaw the worker's injury in the first place, which would mean employers paid the medical costs three times—first, through workers' compensation premiums, second through increased premiums, and third when Social Security requested reimbursement for medical care given to the injured worker.

The consignment of all these RSI sufferers to retirement might not seem so bad when the latest data suggests most of them are middle-aged. But what about when teens begin entering the workforce already injured? If we apply the earlier statistic that predicts a 50 percent higher rate of injured workers among tech-savvy teens to Medicare's current 63.2 percent of costs for the disabled, we find that 94.8 percent of Medicare's costs in the future will go toward covering the disabled. That is, of course, if the SSDI program is even around—it's expected to be exhausted by 2015.[16] The combination of retiring such a large segment of the population early and launching already injured teens into the workforce brings us to another trend adding to the perfect storm—a talent crunch.

CATASTROPHIC LOSS OF HUMAN RESOURCES

According to David G. Allen, PhD, of the Society for Human Resource Management, "a talent scarcity is looming."[17] This talent crunch stems from a number of factors—none as critical as the combination of an aging population and declining birthrate. The strategy of offering early retirement as a cost-saving initiative is proving incredibly shortsighted, which makes the way we've handled RSIs downright dangerous. More and more companies find they need intellectual capital to stay on top. That capital comes in the form of human resources. Intellectual capital includes not only patents and a skilled workforce but also old-fashioned know-how. These are intangible assets to be sure, but they add incredible value to a company.

Baruch Lev, a professor of accounting at New York University, says intellectual capital accounts for more than half the market capitalization of America's public companies.[18] Workers with high intellectual capital and type A personalities who bring a wealth of experience with them are driving innovation today, and we rely on them heavily to compete in the global market. They're also the type of workers who develop RSIs.

A study conducted by Kevin A. Hassett and Robert J. Shapiro for the economic advisory firm Sonecon demonstrates just how much people are a part of this equation. Hassett and Shapiro provided the first systematic valuation of intellectual capital in the United States in 2005. They measured patents, copyrights, and "other forms of economic ideas," which at the time they styled as things like databases and business methods. Importantly, everything they measured, save business methods, could arguably stem from more than just brainpower. It is difficult to quantify how much money was made from someone's idea versus the machine or process derived from that idea. In Hassett and Shapiro's estimation, the total value of US intellectual capital in 2005 was $5.0 to $5.5 trillion. They went back and performed that same valuation in 2011, adding "economic competencies" into the definition of intellectual capital, that is, the ability to identify, expand, and exploit business opportunities—clearly a brainpower-sourced talent—rather than technological innovation. By 2011, in their estimation, the total value of US intellectual capital rose to an estimated $14.5 trillion.[19]

Now, I'm no economist or forensic accountant, and it is unclear how much of this growth comes from brainpower alone. Some would argue that all of it does. But when you consider the 5.9 million new disabled workers on the SSDI roles, alongside the $14.5 trillion in intellectual capital, you have to wonder just how much money we've lost by sidelining so many people. Whether you find unconscionable the loss of human dignity or the fact that we're simply flushing our future down the toilet, you'll agree we simply cannot afford to sit back and let another twenty years go by as a whole generation of already injured teens enters the workforce.

Developing nations, our competitors, are facing the same RSI epidemic. Places like India, China, and the countries of the Middle East have the opportunity to avert the RSI disaster we've courted, while we will still be digging ourselves out of the hole. That future does not look good for our competitive edge.

ADDITIONAL COSTS TO EMPLOYERS

Microsoft's 2008 statistic that RSIs cost employers $600 million in lost work hours also fails to take into account the hidden costs of replacing injured workers who have not been returned to the job. Once again, little data exists on this specifically. Lots of studies, however, examine the hidden cost of turnover for employers. Even if your business does not have the accounting capabilities to perform its own in-house audit, a quick review of the research should give you a good idea of how much losing even one worker to RSI is costing or would cost your company.

The research regarding employee turnover focuses on direct costs, how the turnover affects business performance, and the increasing cost of failing to manage turnover rates. Employee departures cost a company time and resources, as well as money. There is an additional factor here, a creep that takes hold as turnover begets turnover, until a company is wasting a tremendous amount of money through loss of employees. Sounds very similar to the spike experienced by risk managers who implement ergonomics programs, doesn't it? Some of these expenses include wages for temporary employees, overtime for employees covering the departed employee's duties, delays in production and services, decreases in product and service quality, lost clients, lost business opportunities, hiring inducements like relocation expenses and signing bonuses, on-the-job training, including supervisor as well as employee time, mentoring, socialization, and decreases in productivity until the replacement masters the job. Direct replacement costs have been calculated to reach as high as 50 or 60 percent of an employee's annual salary.[20] When indirect, hidden costs are added, the total shoots to from 90 to 200 percent of an employee's annual salary.[21]

When it comes to losing an employee to RSI, a few additional expenses should be taken into account, such as purchasing additional ergonomic equipment, work redesign, and the time it takes to determine whether that employee can continue to do the same job and, if so, how long before he or she is back up to speed. Clearly it is cheaper not to lose your employees to RSIs in the first place; however, the value of an injured employee's intellectual capital also comes into play in determining the expense of replacing versus rehabilitating that worker.

In 1998, Ernst and Young was losing 22 percent of its women professionals at a cost of $150,000 per employee.[22] A mission-critical employee of a California aerospace company developed a disabling RSI and was rushed back to work before she was ready. How much did permanently losing that employee cost that company? This clearly shortsighted error was no doubt caused by the time crunch of the particular mission the company was then engaged in. Wouldn't you rather conduct this survey of how much it's costing your company not to return its injured workers to the job outside the heat of a crisis? In determining how much intellectual capital a particular employee brings to a company, that employee will probably have a better idea then the business owner. As a temporary secretary for twenty years, I can tell you that I often walked into a company reeling in shock as it realized how much its entire operation depended on one person. And that person is never the one anyone would have identified before the employee left.

Turnover is much harder on small businesses, so a cost-benefit analysis would calculate the loss of an injured worker as a ratio to overall company revenues rather than turnover costs alone. Some additional considerations include organizational structures where only one employee has a particular skill or knowledge set, a tighter-knit company culture where one employee injury can cause a spike in other injuries, a smaller pool of in-house replacement workers, having only a few customers or clients who generate the majority of the business, and availability of fewer financial resources to cover replacement costs.

For employers weighing their options in returning an injured employee to work, Manpower's white paper "Confronting the Talent Crunch: 2008" provides some suggestions via retaining retirees and their intellectual capital. Offer them less stressful and time-consuming roles that allow them to share their knowledge and skills in a broader capacity. Some applications include the training of new talent, documenting important information and processes, and acting in a problem-solving capacity. [23]

Talent-management strategies have become a high priority for businesses. Talent-retention programs would require an ergonomics program as well. Research has shown that one of the best ways to retain talent is by building a sense of community within a company's culture. Studies cite "fit"—the main idea behind ergonomics—as key to employees' sense of connection to their companies. A 2008 Ernst and Young study revealed another key talent-retention strategy: respect for work-life balance. Ernst and Young's study cited satisfaction with the workplace environment as the biggest single factor in turnover among key employees. It seems that, in the talent crunch, employers must provide an ergonomics program if they are going to retain the talent necessary to compete in today's marketplace.

ALL THESE COSTS EVENTUALLY RETURN TO WORKERS

When a company has to face paying higher workers' compensation costs and implementing an ergonomics program or closing its doors, you can be sure these costs eventually trickle down to workers in the form of hiring freezes, raise and wage freezes, or extra work. Whether it's increased spending of public funds on disability, lowered per capita tax revenues, or decreased per capita discretionary spending, the cost of RSIs eventually returns to us all.

Instead of contributing to the gross national product, as they once had, RSI sufferers become a drain on our economy. The true cost of that has yet to be calculated.

Chapter Twelve

Why Work Is the Cure for RSIs

Repetitive strain injuries terrify us on a socioeconomic level. They raise questions too uncomfortable to confront. They suggest that we are physically incapable of using the very technology on which we have become dependent. They seem to provide evidence that human beings have a limited capacity for work. They call into question the idea of limitless expansion. Our physical bodies clearly need to catch up, but evolution takes generations. What will happen in the meantime? Can we wait it out? What if we can't use the technology we've developed in the way commerce is driving us to employ it? What if we can't compete in the global marketplace? Are we literally working ourselves and our way of life to death? These questions and anxieties, I believe, have led us to hide RSIs in plain sight.

Ironically, the answers to those questions lie in the very thing we've been trying to bury. Those of us who have learned to live with RSIs have found that they bring a certain wisdom, and despite the terrible pain they have put us through, we recognize in them a gift. An RSI sufferer has to ask, What is health? What is a sustainable lifestyle? How can I still be productive when I have lost significant use of my hands? How can I still contribute? The story of RSIs asks society these same questions.

RSIs call for evolution in how we define and measure work. That evolution is already happening at the theoretical level in academia and among the top-performing companies on the world stage. Instead of having reached a socioeconomic ceiling, we are in fact on the verge of tapping into an entirely new level of human potential. This level has always been there; we've just never valued it before.

HOW WE MEASURE WORK

The thing that drove me most crazy once I became disabled was that I was never able to get anything done. My favorite tool, the to-do list, was always full. Grocery shopping, for instance, had become an endless process entailing no longer just the shopping trip itself but also getting the groceries into the house, and putting the items away. Making meals involved getting those groceries out again, then chopping and preparing before cooking. After I ate, there was the cleanup, then taking the garbage out. Each task was so physically exhausting that I could do only one or two of them in any given day, so that it took me days to complete all the tasks for just one meal. Then the whole, seemingly endless series of tasks started over again. Eventually, however, I realized that rather than just grocery shopping and cooking, I was actually feeding myself. With that shift in perspective, I was easily able to reorganize the job into tasks I could manage.

In 1982, physicist and systems theorist Fritjof Capra predicted this clash between work capacity and output capacity in his book *The Turning Point: Science, Society, and the Rising Culture.* Capra declares that segmented Cartesian thinking can no longer solve society's complex problems and that instead we'll have to employ holism and systems theory.[1] This is what I had to do to resolve the problem of meal preparation. Once I applied a holistic approach, I found ways to make eating more productive; for instance, eating with friends meant I didn't have to handle all the tasks myself, as well as provided society and emotional support from those friends. The same methodology is called for in the way we measure work.

When still an agrarian people, we measured work by harvests yielded. When Henry Ford conceived of the assembly line, he revolutionized our notions about the human capacity to produce, and we began to measure work in terms of goods and services. A similar evolution is happening now as we begin to measure work in terms of intellectual capital. In chapter 11, we saw how much value that adds to our economy. Is it any wonder then that we're now measuring productivity by value received? And interestingly enough, when academics looked for ways to increase value received in terms of productivity, they found some of the same keys necessary to prevent RSIs.

In 1992, Robert Karasek wrote in *Healthy Work: Stress, Productivity, and the Reconstruction of Working Life* that a truer measure of productivity goes beyond output or even profit to include future economic development. To measure that, Karasek developed the idea of the conducive value of output.[2] Conducive value focuses on the growth of skills and capabilities. He examined the implications for productivity, rather than productivity itself. Since previous research already proved a connection between workplace stress and reduced productivity, Karasek placed worker health at the center of his equation. Previous research established two sources for workplace stress: the person and the environment. Because focusing on the person is cheaper and easier, that's where the bulk of science to date has been applied, giving rise to a growing industry of self-help products. Focusing on the environment has been deemed too thorny because doing so would require a total restructuring of workplace control among labor and management. This is the same as the basis of the workers' compensation industry's handling of RSIs —control labor rather than partner with it. Karasek felt this approach only addressed effects, not causes, so he went back to the original workplace stress research.

Research has long concluded that a worker's lack of control in perform- ing a job causes stress. In other words, if the job is psychologically demand- ing but the worker has a great deal of latitude in deciding how to accomplish the tasks required, the resulting job stress is actually low. Conversely, even if the psychological demands of a job are low, if the worker has no decision- making authority in performing tasks, the resulting stress is high. One look at an assembly line easily demonstrates this. The tasks themselves appear to be relatively easy. It's the pressure of performing the tasks under a ticking clock and according to specific, repeated procedures that causes the stress. The actual repetitive motion is just a dramatization of the internal stress the worker is undergoing.

Science long assumed that every job entails an inevitable, immutable set of demands. Karasek removed that assumption. Instead of looking at the output demands of the job, Karasek looked at the organization of individual job tasks. He found that it is "not the demands of work itself, but the organ- izational structure of work, that plays the most consistent role in the develop- ment of stress-related illness."[3] His research revealed further that intellectual capital only truly gets tapped in jobs that give workers wide decision-making latitude, such as managerial and professional occupations, and in jobs that actually push workers beyond their training. He concluded that addressing quality of work life actually increased productivity.

Beginning in 1996, Joseph Kessels, a researcher in human resource devel- opment, began working with a theory he called knowledge productivity, studying "the way in which individuals, teams and units across an organiza- tion achieve knowledge-based improvements and innovations."[4] Under this theory, workers had to be constantly challenged in order to expand their knowledge productivity. This meant that organizations would have to con- stantly challenge their employees in order to glean maximum knowledge productivity. To do that, organizations would have to constantly evolve themselves. Most thought the price too high. Since then, however, this condi- tion of constant challenges has evolved as a consequence of accelerations in technology, necessitating a complete rethinking of literally everything we do in every industry.

The ergonomics programs already described in this book are one example of such knowledge-productivity initiatives. They offer workers growth in skills and capabilities and companies increased performance, as well as create future economic development, which in turn offers more growth in skills and capabilities and an even greater increase in productivity. Employers often confuse job stress with challenge, but meeting a challenge engenders satisfaction; it boosts confidence and actually reduces stress. [5]

WORK REDESIGN

We've already looked at Liberty Mutual's study showing that workspace flexibility and training combined offer the most successful ergonomics programs. But sometimes an ergonomic evaluation reveals that an entire position, process, or even company must be reorganized to reduce workers' physical and psychological stress. This is where workspace flexibility literally means expanding the notions of work and space. This is where a company can really marshal the intellectual capital of its workers, and Karasek's and Kessels's research suggests that although such redesign is challenging, the benefits in growth and productivity are well worth it.

The good news is that you don't have to be a multinational corporation with a billion-dollar restructuring budget to make the jobs in your business more ergonomic and productive. There are small business work-redesign solutions that also happen to be inexpensive. Loss-control consultant Jeff Teideman shares a story about a small guitar-manufacturing company whose employees were experiencing a lot of carpal tunnel–like symptoms, always in the left hand, although all of them were right-handed. The employees all blamed the spray booth part of the operation. Once a guitar is built, it gets sprayed with a protective coating to achieve that beautiful shine. That is done in a spray booth so that dust and other particles do not become embedded in the coating. Teideman asked for a demonstration and saw the problem right away. Workers attached the neck of the guitar to a metal handle, then held the metal handle with their left hand, out to their side, while turning and spraying the guitar. The combination of extending the left arm while holding even such a small amount of weight and twisting the wrist to rotate the guitar was causing the injuries. Teideman worked with the guys in the shop to design a small stand with a rotating clamp that would hold the guitar rather than the workers. Teideman says, "Their guys built the stand, it was very inexpensive, and it completely eliminated the problem." [6]

Ergonomist and epidemiologist Judith Gold shared a similar story, this time involving an auto repair shop. The service technicians cited a particularly difficult repair that required them to crawl under the dashboard, get into an awkward, twisting position, raise their arms above their heads, and then apply torque to operate their tools. This was wreaking havoc on their backs, necks, and wrists. The service technicians themselves engineered a type of creeping platform with two legs on one side and no legs on the other. The platform could be rested against the edge of the car, allowing the mechanic to lie flat, with his arms at head height, not over his head.

Another type of work redesign deals more with organization. As an office worker, I had a great deal of latitude in deciding how to accomplish my assigned tasks. I was the one who had poorly designed my job. I would do all the typing first, then all the photocopying, followed by all the filing. I thought this was a more efficient way to organize the tasks. I could have easily rearranged my work to allow for breaks in the mechanical load by typing one project, then photocopying it, then filing it, followed by the next typing project. I just had no education about the matter.

Gold says that when reorganizing a job, you have to consider what kind of exposure the worker has throughout the day. She offers an example via supposedly ergonomic task rotation on assembly-line jobs. A worker rotates to many different stations on the line, performing different tasks every hour. But, Gold says, if the worker is still using her hands in the same way at each station, that's really not effective from an ergonomic standpoint. "The best kind of job rotations would rotate from the assembly line, to driving a fork-lift, to unpacking supplies," says Gold.[7]

WHAT THIS MEANS FOR THE INDIVIDUAL

The implications of knowledge productivity and conducive value for the individual have the potential to increase personal capital as well. We've already seen how I could have redesigned my own job, without even alerting my employer, which would have saved me a tremendous amount of money. What about applying these same principles to the rest of life? Once I became disabled, I had to reorganize everything I did. I found, for example, that I spent less time running errands on a Tuesday afternoon, when there were fewer people in the stores and fewer cars on the roads, than I did on a Saturday. What if everyone applied these ideas to their lives? What if everyone had more flexible jobs? Could that possibly, say, reduce traffic, a major stressor for all of us?

What strikes me in all these studies is the notion of productive behavior. Organizational psychology defines productive behavior as "behavior that contributes positively to goals and objectives. It promotes, encourages and aids in purpose."[8] If our jobs were the only things stressing us out, we could point to our employers and initiate all those claims the insurance industry is concerned we will file if job stress is definitively linked to illness and injury. But we have to be honest; the rest of our lives are full of stress as well, and there is a lot we can do about that. Again, those of us who battle RSIs have learned to work differently, discovering facilities we never thought we had.

Recall the beautiful music Greg Dempster was able to make after recovering from his RSI. The quality of our lives has improved tremendously. In my case, I look for ways to accomplish things through what I can do and what I'm good at, and I accept that I cannot do everything. When it comes to things I cannot do, I look around me for people who can do them, who are good at them, and who like to do them. Then I trade them what I can do for what they can do. In the end, we're both much happier. It also makes for a far more connected community around me. I would say the quality of our hearts has improved as well. RSIs, in the end, have created tremendous value for us, but only for those of us who have employed the experience and made it work for us.

Our epic Berkeley grad Bonnie says that her decision-making and self-advocacy skills have improved, and for a twenty-five-year-old, that's saying something. In fact, when you meet her, you notice right away that her level of self-awareness far exceeds that of her peers. She calls her internship with the US Department of Labor's Office of Disability Employment Policy (ODEP) an incredible experience. There, she met many people who played significant roles in the disability rights movement, actively contributing to the department's overall mission to improve employment opportunities for all. But she's most excited about the innovative work she participated in as a member of the Youth Policy Team, on which she brought her own experiences reorganizing her life to bear in preparing high school students for college and careers through individualized learning plans. The team studied the results of a US trend in which individual states were implementing legislatively mandated student-directed college- and career-planning programs. "We looked at the strategies that allow youth with disabilities to be successful," Bonnie explained.[9] The team found that youth with disabilities need the same 360 degrees of support that all youth need—including mentoring, recreational opportunities, and work experience—to succeed in college and their careers.

The team also found that static job descriptions are holding students and workers back. Those jobs measure employees' value in direct proportion to their productivity. Bonnie says, "As long as your value to your company is based on your ability to churn out something, we're going to continue to have portions of the population that are excluded."[10] They will then become liabilities to society rather than assets.

The Office of Disability Employment Policy believes everyone has the ability to work—that a doctor's declaration that someone can't erases a huge part of that person's humanity. ODEP likes to focus on harnessing the skills a person can contribute. Bonnie tells the story of one boy with an intellectual disability who was always banging on things with a hammer. He loved to hammer away for hours and hours. The ODEP brought in a job specialist and discovered that this boy liked to build things, so it hired a job coach. The job coach and the boy began to build birdhouses together, which, sure enough, they started selling to the community. The ODEP managed to find a meaningful way for the boy to contribute that gave him a lot of fulfillment.[11]

Clearly, that's a story of going the extra mile, and I'm not advocating instituting that type of proactivity on the institutional level. But we all can apply the same idea at the personal level. We have already looked at the economic cost of allowing such a large portion of our society to become disabled. There is a cost to our overall health as a nation as well. Working gives us so much more than a paycheck.

During my stint in the workers' compensation system and on the board of directors of first the Los Angeles RSI Support Group and then the Cumulative Trauma Disorders Resources Network, I regularly interacted with injured workers. I was most struck by how much we need to work. Yes, those of us who contract RSIs tend to derive far too much meaning in our lives from work, but even the seemingly least motivated person I met in the system, a gas station attendant who was on his third work-related injury, had noticeably lost himself in not being able to work. It made me think a lot about just what work is.

There's a reason we sometimes call work our livelihood. Human beings are herd animals; we need to participate, to contribute to that herd, to feel secure as a part of it. Add sapience, and you begin to see what is possible in terms of our production capacities: we who have developed RSIs and recovered have learned to work smarter, not harder.

In *The Reinvention of Work*, Matthew Fox writes, "A lot of the work in our culture is not paid: raising children, repairing your home, listening to a neighbor. These jobs are important because they put us in touch with our community."[12] If we were to harness not only our knowledge capital but also our human capital, what type of productivity could we then achieve? Research shows that in order to perform at their maximum productivity levels, humans need to use all of their skills, not just some. I believe stress at work comes from not being able to do just that. We're underutilizing our workforce in the name of completing manual tasks that we've already developed technologies to do in our stead. What's lagging is our minds.

Unfortunately, our educational system has not prepared us for this at all. Nor is it preparing the next generation that is about to enter the workforce already injured. Bonnie describes our educational system as "very individualistic and very selfish. It's all about me and my learning. I want my work to contribute to something bigger than me."[13] I think the biggest deficit in our educational system lies in a failure to encourage creative thinking, a skill crucial not only to preventing RSIs but to solving any complex problem before us. My favorite creative-thinking tactic is to make a list of all possible solutions, including the most improbable ones, then to start with the latter and work backward.

Appendix A

Patient Resources

Visual and other resources are available on this book's companion website at http://www.truthaboutcarpaltunnel.com. I offer my RSI coping strategy here by way of example only.

STRATEGIES FOR COPING WITH RSI

To Regain Physical Health

- Get educated on the topic.
- Compare the research to your own experiences.
- Locate health-care practitioners in the disciplines that make sense to you.
- Assemble a team of practitioners, in both traditional and nontraditional disciplines, willing to work with you and each other toward your recovery.
- Maintain pain and functionality logs.
- Share those logs with each and every practitioner, as well as your legal team.
- Make sure your logs become part of your medical record.
- Partner with your practitioners to track your progress.
- Stick with what works; drop what doesn't.
- Make finding a way to remain positive a priority.
- Commit to maintaining your health.

To Address Lifestyle Issues

- Employers, family members, and friends

  - Explain your condition.
  - Offer educational references.
  - Share your recovery plans with them.
  - Provide regular updates on any improvements.
  - Accept all the help offered.
  - Allow friends and family to participate in your plans.
  - Work with friends and family to devise ways to maintain your positive outlook.
  - Work with friends and family to address your mental well-being.

- Work-arounds

  - Make a list of every day tasks you can no longer complete on your own.
  - Share that list with your medical and legal team, as well as family and friends.
  - Ask for ideas about how to approach these tasks for your greatest success and mental well-being.
  - Ask for help where you need it.
  - Make sure you find ways to perform some of those tasks on your own! It'll help build your confidence.

To Return to Work

- Begin with daily activities at home.
- Build a log of tasks and activities from your lifestyle work-around plan.
- Track what you can do over time.
- Work with your medical team to ascertain what types of work activities you can do based on those lifestyle tasks and activities.
- Work with your employer to redesign your job so that you can perform as much of it as possible.
- Work with available career counselors through workers' compensation, disability advocacy groups, and Social Security Disability to identify any new jobs or careers you may be able to do.
- Create a return-to-work plan with all stakeholders.

FINDING A DOCTOR

Optimally, you will find a practitioner who is well versed in RSIs, has seen a lot of patients, and understands what it takes to get you back to work. When looking for a new practitioner, before making the first appointment, call the office and ask the following:

How many RSI patients has the doctor seen?
What training has the doctor had in treating RSIs?
What was the most recent RSI training the doctor received?
What types of diagnostics does the doctor perform on RSI patients?
To what types of specialists does the doctor usually refer RSI patients?
How does the doctor's office work with employers, caregivers, insurers, and legal teams?
What types of programs does the doctor's office have for return-to-work plans?

GETTING AN ACCURATE DIAGNOSIS

Several RSI patient websites under the "Websites" section below describe the most popular, as well as the most effective, testing protocols. Familiarize yourself with the pros and cons of each so that you can discuss your test results from an informed position. Keeping pain and functionality logs will help you get an accurate diagnosis. Once you identify the type of pain and its location, you can select the type of practitioner with whom you will likely have the most success. In addition to the ones already presented in the book, below are the most popular options. Again, these are not presented as medical advice. They're just definitions.

Types of Practitioners to Consider

- Neurologists: Neurologists treat diseases and disorders of the nervous system. They are particularly helpful when experienced in treating RSIs because they can identify difficult-to-diagnose problems. They are also more familiar with centralized pain.
- Occupational physicians: These clinicians work with health and safety in the workplace. Their training includes prevention, epidemiology, and rehabilitation. Anyone in occupational medicine should be extremely familiar with RSIs.
- Osteopaths: Osteopaths are alternative medical doctors who focus on functionality and health. They look to strengthen the musculoskeletal system and take a holistic approach to RSIs.

- Pediatric orthopedists: Orthopedists study the bones, joints, and muscles. Some are surgeons; some are not. They usually specialize in a specific body part, and so often do not take a holistic approach. If you are under age twenty-five, you might consider consulting a pediatric orthopedist with an additional specialization in growing bones and muscles. This is a relatively new field, and information regarding how many RSIs they see is currently unavailable.
- Physiatrists: Physiatrists are rehabilitation specialists. They work with bones, muscles, and nerves, with an emphasis on functionality and movement. They also take a holistic approach, work with other disciplines, and use nonsurgical interventions.
- Psychologists/psychiatrists: RSI is extremely tough to deal with on a psychological level. Constant or chronic pain causes substantial changes in the body's chemistry that researchers don't yet understand. Don't be shy!
- Rheumatologists: Rheumatologists are trained in illness rather than injury, with particular familiarity with complex diseases. They also have training in the musculoskeletal system and pain, and their work often involves the internal organs as well.

Treatment Methods to Consider

- Alexander technique: The Alexander technique, a movement awareness practice, was originally developed to help artists and performers. It features work with a practitioner or self-study materials available at http://www.alexandertechnique.com.
- Behavioral modification therapy: Behavior modification therapy focuses on what you do and how you do it; talk therapy focuses more on why you do it. I found this type of therapy very helpful in tackling the sleep disorder. It is also quite useful in discerning progress.
- Egoscue method: Egoscue is a method of postural retraining that many RSI sufferers have had success with. You can find more information at http://www.egoscue.com.
- Feldenkreis: This is a movement-retraining discipline that uses somatics. In addition to classes with a trained practitioner, several audio and video products are available. For more information, visit http://achievingexcellence.com.
- Pain management: Pain management specialists are there to help you deal with your pain. Be careful that the clinic uses a multidisciplinary approach that includes nonpharmaceuticals, nutrition, exercise, and mental well-being.

TOOLS

The American Chronic Pain Association's website has terrific communication tools (http://theacpa.org/Communication-Tools). They include pain diagrams, pain logs, functionality charts, a quality-of-life scale, daily activity checklists, a tool for preparing for your first doctor's visit, and a fibro log.

SUPPORT GROUPS

There are numerous support groups around the globe. A few are listed blow. See the "Websites" section for sites with a more extensive list of support groups.

East Bay RSI is a large and very involved community (http://www. meetup.com/rsi-2).

The Sorehands Listserv is a good place to find fellow sufferers, get specific questions answered, and pole the community on ergonomic products. Sign up by sending an e-mail to listserv@listsrv.ucsf.edu.

The Typing Injury Frequently Asked Questions website provides an exhaustive listing of support group links and evaluations of ergonomic products (http://www.tifaq.com).

ERGONOMIC PRODUCTS

When looking for an ergonomics product, read product reviews, talk to people who use the product, and then try it out for yourself. A good place to start is the National Ergonomics Conference and ErgoExpo (http://www. ergoexpo.com). Even if you can't attend, the website contains a list of exhibitors from current years.

RECOMMENDED READING

Conquering Carpal Tunnel Syndrome, by Sharon Butler, April 1996

Dr. Pascarelli's Complete Guide to Repetitive Strain Injury: What You Need to Know about RSI and Carpal Tunnel, by Emil Pascarelli, MD, 2004

Job's Body, by Deane Juhan, 2003

"Piano School Tones Up the Hands on the Keys," *New York Times,* 1986 (http://www.nytimes.com/1986/07/27/arts/piano-school-tones-up-the-hands-on-the-keys.html)

Repetitive Strain Injury: A Computer User's Guide, by Emil Pascarelli, MD, and Deborah Quilter, 1994

"Thoracic Outlet Syndrome (TOS) Information," by Dr. James D. Collins, Radiologist, UCLA (http://tosinfo.com)

TYPING RETRAINING

Greg Dempster's typing retraining website is at www.triangleassociates-us.com.

VIDEOS

"3D CGI Medical Video Carpal Tunnel Syndrome," http://www.youtube.come/watch?v=u5dwtGYQ6PU.

"Amy Cuddy: Your Body Language Shapes Who You Are," TED, October 2012 (www.ted.com/talks/amy_cuddy_your_body_language_shapes_who_you_are.html)

"Better Health with 5 Breaths a Day!" by Smokin Yogi, YouTube, March 9, 2009 (http://www.youtube.com/watch?v=gMwXUuIU34M)

"Elliot Krane: The Mystery of Chronic Pain," TED, May 2011 (http://www.ted.com/talks/elliot_krane_the_mystery_of_chronic_pain.html)

"Forward Head Posture Correction (Anti-Ageing Must)," by Posturevideos.com, YouTube, June 8, 2011 (http://www.youtube.com/watch?v=4uzd_nFzj0Y)

"Nociceptive and Neuropathic Pain.mpg," by Lynne Columbus, YouTube, April 15, 2012 (www.youtube.com/watch?v=sg2y34hmEew)

"Yoga Nidra" (guided relaxation meditation), , YouTube, September 8, 2013 (http://www.youtube.com/watch?v=vvldC6mzLvA)

Tibetan singing bowl meditations, Brian Green (http://seeyouinsleep.com/store)

WEBSITES

The RSI community is very good about sharing vetted information. I recommend you start with organization-based sites first.

The RSI information page at the University of Michigan has good descriptions of risk factors, workstation setup, and prevention exercises (http://web.eecs.umich.edu/~cscott/rsi.html).

The website of the RSI and Overuse Injury Association of the ACT provides lots of practical information on all aspects of RSI for the patient. The work-arounds section is extensive. The association also publishes a lively and informative newsletter (http://www.rsi.org.au).

UCLA's ergonomics page has some good posture strengthening exercises and stretches for multiple body areas (http://ergonomics.ucla.edu/component/content/article/83-injuries-and-prevention/111-repetitive-strain-injury-rsi).

RSI Action is sponsored by the Massachusetts Coalition for Occupational Safety and Health. Its website is information laden with lots of links (http://www.rsiaction.org).

Sharon Butler is a Hellerworker practitioner and carpal tunnel sufferer. Her website has prevention information, exercises, and stretches (http://www.selfcare4rsi.com). Her book, *Conquering Carpal Tunnel Syndrome*, is considered the gold standard in self-care.

Paul Marxhausen's website has good pictures and videos of exercises, as well as a good list of RSI books (http://rsi.unl.edu).

Scriven's "RSI-Related Resources" page has some Dragon NaturallySpeaking macros (http://www.scriven.com/RSI/RSIdata/rsidata.html).

MIT has an RSI prevention page (http://web.mit.edu/atic/www/rsi/index.html).

Appendix B

Parent Resources

While the research on teens and texting is still in its nascent stages, it doesn't take a social scientist to recognize that, as children hit puberty, a strong confluence of influences makes for awkwardness while they begin the process of developing into adults. It is easy to hide in technology as a way of coping with this awkwardness. Therefore, it is important for parents to help their children develop a sense of self outside that technology by helping them develop the social skills that will allow them to both express their individuality and find their natural confidence. These tools are also very good for adults who have become addicted to their technology!

DEVELOPING A SENSE OF SELF

"Presentation of Self on the Web: An Ethnographic Study of Teenage Girls' Weblogs," by Denise Sevick Bortree, Paul Dowling's Website, March 2005 (www.pauldowling.me/r%26d/papers/bortree(2005).pdf)

"The Consciousness Question: Nature, Nurture, and the Hundred Billion Neurons in Between," by Graham Collier, *Psychology Today*, December 21, 2011 (www.psychologytoday.com/blog/the-consciousness-question/201112/sense-self)

"It's So Hard to Be Your Friend: Teaching Social Skills to Teens," Clinton Smith, EdD, and Kay Reeves, EdD, University of Memphis (https://umdrive.memphis.edu/csmith15/public/It's%20So%20Hard%20to%20be%20Your%20Friend.pdf).

The Friendship Circle website has "12 Activities to help your child with social skills" (www.Friendshipcircle.org). Although these activities are meant as special-needs resources, they also provide great ways for parents to think of helping their teens develop better social skills.

Believe it or not, games for actors are perfect for helping to develop crucial social skills, especially listening and responding. Improvisational games are also a lot of fun and can replace charades at family game night. An excellent online source for these includes http://www.ace-your-audition.com/acting-exercises.html. Drama Resources has some terrific games the whole family can play at http://dramaresource.com/games. Improve Encyclopedia has enough games to keep you busy at http://improvencyclopedia.org/games.

The National Institutes of Health have some very good supplemental curriculum materials available on its website, including lesson plans and interactive activities.

- "The Brain: Our Sense of Self, NIH Curriculum Supplement Series—Grades 7–8" (http://science.education.nih.gov/supplements/nih4/self/default.htm)
- "The Science of Healthy Behavior, NIH Curriculum Supplement Series—Grades 7–8" (http://science.education.nih.gov/supplements/nih7/healthy/default.htm)
- "The Science of Energy Balance: Calorie Intake and Physical Activity, NIH Curriculum Supplement Series—Grades 7–8" (http://science.education.nih.gov/supplements/nih4/Energy/default.htm)

"Film Legend Herzog Takes on Texting and Driving," Todd Leopold, CNN, August 16, 2013 (http://www.cnn.com/2013/08/16/tech/mobile/werner-herzog-texting-driving)

HOLDING A FAMILY MEETING

Present the information on RSIs to everyone in the family. Agree to set limits on technology usage for the whole family. Golden Path Games has an excellent workbook on how to hold a family meeting at http://creativetherapytechniques.weebly.com/uploads/2/3/7/7/2377039/_family_meeting_materials_for_copying.pdf

CONTROLLING THE AMOUNT OF TEXTING

You can limit the amount of texting and to whom on most phones through the "parental controls" function. The Teen Safe mobile app allows you to track your teens' texting habits if you and/or your teen can't adhere to the agreed-on limits (https://cp.teensafe.com/?sid=1002&cid=14&aff_sub=102315fe6a2e0e187dbeafd97cfea7).

Cafemom.com has some practical tips (http://www.cafemom.com/advice/teens/technology/180/How_can_I_limit_my_teens_texting).

The Mayo Clinic has tips for setting and monitoring texting limits (http://www.mayoclinic.com/health/teen-texting/MY00936).

ILPS

For students, an ILP is an individualized learning plan; for adults in career transition, an ILP is an integrated life plan. Either way, an ILP is an excellent tool for developing and maintaining focus on goals. Students are using ILPs to prepare themselves for college, the disabled use them to plan for returning to work, and adults transitioning through career changes also use them. Several already include health goals, but since all of these are modular, it's easy to add health goals into an overall plan.

The National Collaborative on Workforce and Disability's ILP planning tools are excellent for focusing youth on entering the workforce; they include planning tools, videos, podcasts, and resources broken down by overall goals (http://www.ncwd-youth.info/ilp/how-to-guide).

The American Youth Policy Forum's website has a video with complete instructions for preparing such a plan (http://www.aypf.org/resources/the-use-of-individualized-learning-plans-to-help-students-to-be-college-and-career-ready-2).

"Realize Your Dreams with a Life Plan" by eLifePlans.com is more for adults; it provides step-by-step directions on how to create an ILP (http://www.elifeplans.com/helpful/lifeplanseminardownload.pdf).

Dreamweavers Institute talks about life's chapters on its website for developing a meaningful life. The first chapter discusses the twenties, a time when an individual desires to leave home and begin his or her individual life. The focus is on increasing responsibility while avoiding commitments and keeping options open for exploration (http://www.dreamweaversinstitute.com/resources.htm).

Appendix C

Employer Resources

Your best place to find resources is your workers' compensation insurance carrier. Some states require by law that workers' compensation insurers provide loss-prevention services. Check your state's insurance department website for more information. If you have a workers' compensation insurance policy, contact your carrier's loss-prevention department to see what programs it has available.

CLAIMS MANAGEMENT RESOURCES

HUB International has a good presentation on employer claims management at www.hubinternational.com/uploadedfiles/corporate/webinars/risk_services/wc%20claims%20management%20webinar%20-%209-13-12.pdf.

"Managing Workers' Compensation Claims," by Philip E. Goldsmith, CSP, ARM, is good on effective claims management (http://www.asse.org/practicespecialties/riskmanagement/docs/Goldsmith%20Paper.pdf).

M3 Insurance provides a good, visually laden plan for claims management (http://m3ins.com/assets/documents-pdfs/ARTICLE_Managing_WC_Claims.pdf)

RETURN-TO-WORK PROGRAMS

The New York Workers' Compensation Board has a good return-to-work brochure at www.wcb.ny.gov/content/main/ReturnToWork/RTW_ Handbook.pdf.

The Risk Institute has a terrific presentation on return-to-work programs that debunks a lot of myths and demonstrates the benefits of a good program (www.riskinstitute.org/peri/images/file/FPSH_Chapter_1_ RTW_206.pdf).

IMPLEMENTING AN ERGONOMICS PROGRAM

A comprehensive definition of the types of ergonomics helps employers understand the scope of the issues when considering health and safety programs for their companies. According to the International Ergonomics Association, other considerations include cognitive ergonomics (perception, memory, reasoning, motor response, human-computer interaction, mental workloads, decision making, skilled performance, human reliability, work stress, training, and user experiences); organizational ergonomics (communication, crew resource management, work design, schedules, teamwork, participation, community, cooperative work, new work programs, virtual organizations, and telework); and environmental ergonomics (climate, temperature, pressure, vibration, and light).

The Centers for Disease Control and the National Institute of Occupational Safety and Health have excellent materials on workplace stress, including definitions, examples, points of discussion, and a step-by-step guide at http://www.cdc.gov/niosh/docs/99-101.

The Occupational Safety and Health Administration's website contains workstation-evaluation guidelines, checklists, and work-process evaluations at https://www.osha.gov/SLTC/etools/computerworkstations/ workprocess.html.

The State Compensation Insurance Fund of California has a sample ergonomics program on its website at www.statefundca.com/pdf/ sftySampleProg.rtf.

Jonathan Bailin has excellent pictures, FAQs, and comprehensive discussion on creating a healthy workplace at http://www.ergonomicsdr. com/ergonomicsdr.com/ErgonomicsDR.html.

See "Office Ergonomics: Practical Solutions for a Safer Workplace," by WISHA Services Division, Washington State Department of Labor and Industries (http://www.lni.wa.gov/IPUB/417-133-000.pdf).

JOB REDESIGN

"Beyond Top-Down and Bottom-Up Work Redesign: Customizing Job
Content through Idiosyncratic Deals," Severin Hornung, Denise M.
Rousseau, Jürgen Glaser, Peter Angerer, and Matthias Weigl. *Journal
of Organizational Behavior* 31 (2010): 187–215 (http://homepages.se.
edu/cvonbergen/files/2013/01/Beyond-top-down-and-bottom-up-
work-redesign_Customizing-job-content-through-idiosyncratic-deals.
pdf)

"Workplace Redesign: Flexibility, Customization Can Help Employers
Meet Their Bottom Line," by Jacquelyn Flowers, 2008 (www.google.
com/url?sa=t&rct=j&q=&esrc=s&source=web&cd=7&ved=
0CFYQFjAG&url=http%3A%2F%2Fwww.dol.
gov%2Fodep%2Fdocuments%2F09b79519_052c_4c6d_abc6_
3afb0a285baa.doc&ei=STOVUqjhEpTcoASXhYJA&usg=
AFQjCNFxH1_Te1QAdu824s22-vr7y4TlWg&bvm=bv.57155469,d.
cGU).

TYPING RETRAINING

Greg Dempster's typing retraining website is at www.triangleassociates-
us.com.

Notes

1. I WOKE UP ONE MORNING TO FIND MY LIFE HAD FALLEN APART

1. Gavin DeBecker, *The Gift of Fear: Survival Signals That Protect Us from Violence* (Boston: Little, Brown, 1997), 75.

2. WHY IT'S IMPORTANT TO EDUCATE YOURSELF ABOUT RSIS

1. Peter Mandel, MD, comment made at US Department of Labor, Public Forums on Ergonomics, Stanford University, California, July 24, 2001.

2. "Computer Usage in the U.S.," Pew Internet and American Life Project Tracking Survey, December 2008, accessed May 26, 2012, http://www.infoplease.com/ipa/A0921872.html#ixzz1w0G4V2I5.

3. Aaron Smith, "35 Percent of American Adults Own a Smartphone," Pew Internet Project, July 11, 2011, accessed May 26, 2012, http://pewInternet.org/~/media//Files/Reports/2011/PIP_Smartphones.pdf.

4. Aaron Smith, "Mobile Access 2010," Pew Internet Project, July 7, 2010, accessed May 26, 2012, http://www.pewInternet.org/~/media/Files/Reports/2010/PIP_Mobile_Access_2010.pdf.

5. Kristen Purcell, "E-Reader Ownership Doubles in Six Months," Pew Internet Project, June 27, 2011, accessed May 26, 2012, http://pewInternet.org/~/media/Files/Reports/2011/PIP_eReader_Tablet.pdf.

6. Victoria J. Rideout, Ulla G. Foehr, and Donald F. Roberts, "Generation M2: Media in the Lives of 8 to 18 Year Olds," Kaiser Family Foundation, January 2010, accessed January 20, 2014, http://files.eric.ed.gov/fulltext/ED527859.pdf.

7. Adam Daley, "CDC Survey: Carpal Tunnel Syndrome Mostly Linked to Work," MedicalDaily.com, December 23, 2011, http://www.medicaldaily.com/cdc-survey-carpal-tunnel-syndrome-mostly-linked-work-239127.

8. Walter F. Stewart et al., "Lost Productive Time and Cost Due to Common Pain Conditions in the US Workforce," *JAMA* 290, no. 18 (2003): 2443–54, accessed May 27, 2012, doi: 10.1001/jama.290.18.2443.

9. "Carpal Tunnel Syndrome," *New York Times*, February 17, 2011, accessed May 26, 2012, http://health.nytimes.com/health/guides/disease/carpal-tunnel-syndrome/prognosis.html.

10. Paul Dougherty, "Public Health, Musculoskeletal Disorders and Chiropractic: The Time Is Now," American Public Health Association, fall 2009, accessed May 26, 2012, http://www.apha.org/membergroups/newsletters/sectionnewsletters/chiro/fall09/doughtery.htm.

11. Dino Drudi, "Brief: Have Disorders Associated with Repeated Trauma Stopped Increasing?" Bureau of Labor Statistics, summer 2007, accessed January 20, 2014, http://www.bls.gov/opub/mlr/cwc/have-disorders-associated-with-repeated-trauma-stopped-increasing.pdf.

12. Jonathan Bailin, telephone interview with author, Austin, Texas, June 14, 2013.

13. "Carpal Tunnel Syndrome."

14. Bailin, telephone interview.

15. David A. Williams, PhD, telephone interview with author, Austin, Texas, July 9, 2013.

16. Williams, telephone interview.

17. Lauretta Claussen, "Workplace Myth? Carpal Tunnel Syndrome from Computer Use Unlikely, Experts Claim," *Safety and Health Magazine*, October 1, 2011, accessed November 18, 2013, http://www.safetyandhealthmagazine.com/articles/6383-workplace-myth.

18. George J. Piligian, MD, telephone interview with author, Austin, Texas, August 11, 2013.

19. Piligian, telephone interview.

20. Atul Gawande, "How Do We Heal Medicine?" TED, April 2012, http://www.ted.com/talks/atul_gawande_how_do_we_heal_medicine.html.

21. Penney Cowan, telephone interview with author, Austin, Texas, July 2, 2013.

22. S. E. Luckhaupt et al., "Prevalence and Work-Relatedness of Carpal Tunnel Syndrome in the Working Population," 2010 National Health Interview Survey, *American Journal of Industrial Medicine*, accessed May 26, 2012, doi: 10.1002/ajim.22048.

23. Bailin, telephone interview.

24. Gowan, telephone interview.

3. HOW CAN YOU BECOME DISABLED JUST BY SITTING AT A COMPUTER?

1. George J. Piligian, MD, telephone interview with author, Austin, Texas, August 13, 2013.

2. Peter I. Edgelow, "A New Perspective on the Etiology, Evaluation and Management of Patients with Signs and Symptoms of Chronic Pain and Cumulative Trauma Disorder" (presented at the Los Angeles Repetitive Strain Injury Support Group, Wellspring Therapy Clinic, Glendale, California, October 2000).

3. Piligian, telephone interview.

4. Bernard J. Healey and Kenneth T. Walker, *Introduction to Occupational Health in Public Health Practice* (New York: Wiley and Sons, 2009).

5. N. R. Sims and H. Muyderman, "Mitochondria, Oxidative Metabolism and Cell Death in Stroke," *Biochimica et Biophysica Acta* 1802, no. 1 (January 2010): 80–91.

6. "Occupational Overuse Syndrome," XTRA: Health: A–Z of Health, January 3, 2001, accessed October 8, 2001, http://222.xtra.co.nz/health/0,,747-38487,00.html.

7. "New Jersey Spine and Rehabilitation," last modified 2012, http://askthetrucker.com/increase-in-spinal-back-pain-among-long-haul-truck-drivers.

8. Emil Pascarelli and Deborah Quilter, *Repetitive Strain Injury: A Computer User's Guide* (New York: Wiley, 1994), 30.

9. Shelly Atwood, telephone interview with author, Austin, Texas, September 15, 2013.

10. Atwood, telephone interview.

11. Ann Cuddy, "Your Body Language Shapes Who You Are," TED, October 2012, http://www.ted.com/talks/amy_cuddy_your_body_language_shapes_who_you_are.html.

12. Lamar Bush, in-person interview with author, Austin, Texas, June 3, 2013.

13. Bush, in-person interview.

14. Deane Juhan, *Job's Body: A Handbook for Bodywork* (Barrytown, NY: Barrytown, 1998), 86.

15. Juhan, *Job's Body*, 63–86.

16. Juhan, *Job's Body*, 86.

17. Juhan, *Job's Body*, 86.

18. Edgelow, "A New Perspective"

19. R. D. Lockhart, G. F. Hamilton, and F. W. Fyfe, *Anatomy of the Human Body*, (Philadelphia: J. B. Lippincott, 1965), 152.

20. Juhan, *Job's Body*, 184–85.

21. Amanda Lenhart, "Teens, Smartphones & Texting," Pew Research Center's Internet and American Life Project, March 19, 2012, accessed January 20, 2014, http://www.pewinternet.org/~/media/Files/Reports/2012/PIP_Teens_Smartphones_and_Texting.pdf.

22. Ki Mae Heussner, "Teen Gets Carpal Tunnel from Texting," ABC News, March 19, 2010, http://abcnews.go.com/Technology/teen-carpal-tunnel-texting/story?id=10146773.

23. That is, 160 characters per text at 3 ounces of force per key equals 480 ounces of force, or 30 pounds, per text.

24. Victoria J. Rideout, Ulla G. Foehr, and Donald F. Roberts, "Generation M2: Media in the Lives of 8 to 18 Year Olds," Kaiser Family Foundation, January 2010, accessed January 20, 2014, http://files.eric.ed.gov/fulltext/ED527859.pdf.

25. Rideout, Foehr, and Roberts, "Generation M2."

26. Juhan, *Job's Body*, 136–37.

4. WHEN YOU DON'T GET PROPER TREATMENT, YOUR RSI GETS WORSE

1. Giresh Kanji, "The Flight/Fight Response in Chronic Pain," Southern Cross Hospital, http://sportsandpain.co.nz/painclinic/wp-content/uploads/2012/04/Advice-sheet-adrenaline.pdf.

2. Kanji, "The Flight/Fight Response."

3. R. S. Stewart et al., "Cerebral Blood Flow Changes during Sodium-Lactate-Induced Panic Attacks," *American Journal of Psychiatry* 145, no. 4 (April 1988): 442–49.

4. David A. Williams, PhD, telephone interview with author, Austin, Texas, July 9, 2013.

5. Williams, telephone interview.

6. Williams, telephone interview.

7. Williams, telephone interview.

8. Williams, telephone interview.

9. Williams, telephone interview.

10. Williams, telephone interview.

11. N. K. Y. Tang and C. Crane, "Suicidality in Chronic Pain: A Review of the Prevalence, Risk Factors and Psychological Links," *Psychological Medicine* 36 (2006): 575–86, doi: 10.1017/S0033291705006859.

5. ERGONOMICS ALONE CANNOT PREVENT RSIS

1. "What Is Ergonomics?" International Ergonomics Association, 2000, accessed January 20, 2014, http://www.iea.cc/whats/index.html.
2. Greg Dempster, telephone interview with author, Austin, Texas, August 8, 2013.
3. Dempster, telephone interview.
4. Dempster, telephone interview.
5. Dempster, telephone interview.
6. Dempster, telephone interview.
7. Dempster, telephone interview.
8. Jonathan Bailin, telephone interview with author, Austin, Texas, June 24, 2013.
9. Bailin, telephone interview.
10. Berit Schiottz-Christensen et al., "The Role of Active Release Manual Therapy for Upper Extremity Overuse Syndromes—a Preliminary Report," *Journal of Occupational Rehabilitation* 9, no. 3 (September 1999): 201–11.
11. Lamar Bush, in-person interview with author, Austin, Texas, June 3, 2013.
12. David A. Williams, PhD, telephone interview with author, Austin, Texas, July 9, 2013.
13. Marian S. Garfinkel, EdD, telephone interview with author, Austin, Texas, September 9, 2013.
14. Marian S. Garfinkel et al., "Yoga-Based Intervention for Carpal Tunnel Syndrome: A Randomized Trial," *JAMA* 280, no. 18 (1998): 1601–3, doi: 10.1001/jama.280.18.1601.
15. Garfinkel, telephone interview.
16. Garfinkel, telephone interview.

6. WHY THE HEALTH-CARE COMMUNITY DISPUTES THE EXISTENCE OF RSIS

1. Paul Dougherty, "Public Health, Musculoskeletal Disorders and Chiropractic: The Time Is Now," American Public Health Association, fall 2009, accessed May 26, 2012. http://www.apha.org/membergroups/newsletters/sectionnewsletters/chiro/fall09/doughtery.htm.
2. Lauretta Claussen, "Workplace Myth? Carpal Tunnel Syndrome from Computer Use Unlikely, Experts Claim," *Safety and Health Magazine*, October 1, 2011, accessed November 18, 2013, http://www.safetyandhealthmagazine.com/articles/6383-workplace-myth.
3. Judith Gold, Skype interview with author, Austin, Texas, July 30, 2013.
4. Washington Health Policy Fellows, "Musculoskeletal Education in Medical Schools: Are We Making the Cut?" American Association of Orthopaedic Surgeons, March–April 2007, http://www.aaos.org/news/bulletin/marapr07/reimbursement2.asp.
5. Washington Health Policy Fellows, "Musculoskeletal Education in Medical Schools."
6. George J. Piligian, MD, telephone interview with author, Austin, Texas, August 11, 2013.
7. Piligian, telephone interview, August 11, 2013.
8. James D. Collins, MD, telephone interview with author, Austin, Texas, August 5, 2013.
9. Collins, telephone interview.
10. I. Ibrahim et al., "Carpal Tunnel Syndrome: A Review of the Recent Literature," *Open Orthopaedics Journal* 6 (2012): 69–76.
11. Collins, telephone interview.
12. Collins, telephone interview.
13. Collins, telephone interview.
14. Mónica López-Alonso et al., "The Health Effects of Vibrations on the Upper Extremities of Workers" (prepared for the Global Virtual Conference, University of Granada, Department of Projects and Construction Engineering, April 8–12, 2013).

15. George J. Piligian, MD, telephone interview with author, Los Angeles, California, November 17, 2013.

16. Collins, telephone interview.

17. Piligian, telephone interview, November 17, 2013.

18. American Academy of Orthopaedic Surgeons (AAOS), "AAOS Clinical Guidelines on the Treatment of Carpal Tunnel Syndrome," *AAOS Now*, October 2008, http://www.aaos.org/news/aaosnow/oct08/clinical3.asp.

19. New York State Workers' Compensation Board, *New York Carpal Tunnel Syndrome Medical Treatment Guidelines* (New York: New York Workers' State Compensation Board, 2013), 3.

20. Robert Pear, "Percentage of Americans Lacking Health Coverage Falls Again," *New York Times*, September 17, 2013, http://www.nytimes.com/2013/09/18/us/percentage-of-americans-lacking-health-coverage-falls-again.html?_r=0.

7. HOW THE WORKERS' COMPENSATION SYSTEM WORSENS RSIS

1. Adam Daley, "CDC Survey: Carpal Tunnel Syndrome Mostly Linked to Work," MedicalDaily.com, December 23, 2011, http://www.medicaldaily.com/cdc-survey-carpal-tunnel-syndrome-mostly-linked-work-239127.

2. Paul B. Bellamy, *A History of Workmen's Compensation, 1898–1915: From Courtroom to Boardroom* (New York and London: Garland Publishing, 1997), 148.

3. Christopher A. Ball, *Take Charge of Your Workers' Compensation Claim: An A to Z Guide for Injured Employees*, 2nd ed. (Berkeley, CA: Nolo, 2001), 8/8.

4. "CWCI Scorecard Looks at Carpal Tunnel Claims in California WC," WorkCompWire, January 11, 2013, accessed October 13, 2013, http://www.workcompwire.com/2013/01/cwci-scorecard-looks-at-carpal-tunnel-claims-in-california-wc.

5. "CWCI Scorecard Looks at Carpal Tunnel Claims in California WC."

6. Cathy Stanton, telephone interview with author, Austin, Texas, October 1, 2013.

7. New York State Workers' Compensation Board, *New York Carpal Tunnel Syndrome Medical Treatment Guidelines* (New York: New York Workers' State Compensation Board, 2013).

8. New York State Workers' Compensation Board, *New York Carpal Tunnel Syndrome Medical Treatment Guidelines*.

9. Andrew M. Cuomo, "Governor Cuomo Details Improvements to New York's Workers' Compensation System That Cut Costs to Employers by 26% for 2014," Office of the Governor, Albany, New York, October 30, 2013, https://www.governor.ny.gov/press/10302013-ny-workers-compensation-system.

10. Ishita Sengupta, Marjorie Baldwin, and Virginia Reno, *Workers' Compensation: Benefits, Coverage, and Costs, 2011*, National Academy of Social Insurance, August 2013, accessed January 20, 2014, http://www.nasi.org/research/2013/report-workers-compensation-benefits-coverage-costs-2011.

11. Ted Rohrlich and Evelyn Larrubia, "Public Fraud Unit Favors Those Who Privately Fund It," *Los Angeles Times*, August 6, 2000, http://articles.latimes.com/2000/aug/06/news/mn-65499.

12. Rohrlich and Larrubia, "Public Fraud Unit Favors Those Who Privately Fund It."

13. J. Paul Leigh et al., *Costs of Occupational Injuries and Illnesses* (Ann Arbor: University of Michigan Press, 2000), 195.

14. Rohrlich and Larrubia, "Public Fraud Unit Favors Those Who Privately Fund It."

15. Steve Smith, Richard Gannon, and Peggy Sugarman, *Annual Report for 1998*, California Department of Industrial Relations, Division of Workers' Compensation, accessed April 1, 2002, http://www.dir.ca.gov/DWC/98DWCAR.htm.

16. Don Jergler, "Carriers 'Uncertain' about California Workers' Comp Reform," *Insurance Journal*, December 19, 2012, http://www.insurancejournal.com/news/west/2012/12/19/274774.htm.

17. Lloyd Dixon, James W. Macdonald, and William Barbagallo, "California's Volatile Workers' Compensation Insurance Market: Problems and Recommendations for Change" (prepared for the Commission on Health and Safety and Workers' Compensation, Rand Corporation, Center for Health and Safety in the Workplace and Navigant Consulting, 2009), http://www.dir.ca.gov/chswc/reports/2009/insolvencyreport.pdf.

18. Jeff Teideman, telephone interview with author, Austin, Texas, October 6, 2013.

19. Teideman, telephone interview.

20. California Commission on Health and Safety and Workers' Compensation, *2012 Annual Report*, State of California, Labor and Workforce Development Agency, Department of Industrial Relations, December 2012.

21. California Commission on Health and Safety and Workers' Compensation, *2012 Annual Report*.

22. "Employer and Insurer Fraud: Boosting Bottom Line Profits at the Expense of Workers and Society," Workers Injury Law and Advocacy Group (WILG), October 2011.

23. "Employer and Insurer Fraud."

24. "Employer and Insurer Fraud."

25. Greg Dempster, telephone interview with author, Austin, Texas, August 8, 2013.

26. Dempster, telephone interview.

27. W. Pereira, P. Tittiranonda, and S. Burastero, "Ergonomic Analysis of Movement Retraining of Computer Users: A Pilot Study" (presented at the Triennial IEA/HFES Conference, San Diego, California, August 2000).

28. Dempster, telephone interview.

8. THE POLITICAL BATTLE OVER RSIS

1. Dino Drudi, "Brief: Have Disorders Associated with Repeated Trauma Stopped Increasing?" Bureau of Labor Statistics, summer 2007, accessed January 20, 2014, http://www.bls.gov/opub/mlr/cwc/have-disorders-associated-with-repeated-trauma-stopped-increasing.pdf.

2. Mark A. Spognardi and Staci L. Ketay, "Perspective—Bad Law and Bad Politics: OSHA's Ill-Fated Ergonomics Standard," *Employee Relations Law Journal* 27, no. 1 (summer 2001): 85–90.

3. Gabriele Bammer and Brian Martin, "Repetition Strain Injury in Australia: Medical Knowledge, Social Movement, and De Facto Partisanship," *Social Problems* 39, no. 3 (August 1992): 219–37.

4. Greg Foley, "Occupational Health and Safety in Australian Workplaces—the High Risk and High Cost of Serious Body Stressing Incidents," National and Workplace Statistics and Epidemiology Team, National Occupational Health and Safety Commission, November 1996.

5. *RSI and Overuse Injury Association of the Act, Inc. Newsletter*, ACT Health and the Southern Cross Club, autumn/April 2013.

6. "National OHS Strategy 2002–2012: Priority Mechanism Progress," Safe Work Australia, 2012, http://www.safeworkaustralia.gov.au/sites/SWA/about/Publications/Documents/232/National%20OHS%20Strategy%20Priority%20mechanism%20progress%20factsheet.pdf.

7. "The Cost of Work-Related Injury and Illness for Australian Employers, Workers and the Community 2008–09," Safe Work Australia, 2012, http://www.safeworkaustralia.gov.au/sites/swa/about/publications/pages/cost-injury-illness-2008-09.

8. Phil Hardberger, "Texas Workers' Compensation: A Ten Year Survey—Strengths, Weaknesses, and Recommendations," 32 St. Mary's L.J. 1, 6 (2000).

9. Hardberger, "Texas Workers' Compensation."

10. Gary A. Thornton, "Walmart Opted Out, but the Sky Is Not Falling," *State Bar of Texas Workers' Compensation Section Newsletter* 1, no. 6 (summer 2012), accessed January 20, 2014, http://www.texasworkerscompensationsection.com/Newsletters/summer2012.pdf.

11. Occupational Safety and Health Administration, "Enforcement," OSHA, accessed September 25, 2013, https://www.osha.gov/SLTC/ergonomics/faqs.html.

12. Alexandra Berzon and Melanie Trottman, "OSHA Seeks to Make Injury Records Public," *Wall Street Journal*, November 7, 2013, http://online.wsj.com/news/articles/SB10001424052702304672404579182480900278574.

13. Marla Dickerson, "Chiropractic Claims Pain California Employers," *Los Angeles Times*, August 17, 2003, http://articles.latimes.com/2003/aug/17/business/fi-chiro17.

14. "New Calif. Workers' Comp Law: A Mixed Bag for Chiropractic," ChiroWeb, accessed December 11, 2013, http://www.chiroweb.com/mpacms/dc_ca/article.php?id=46235.

15. Liberty Mutual Research Institute for Safety, "Office Worker Safety: Ergonomic Interventions," *From Research to Reality* 15, no. 1 (summer 2012).

16. Jay Bradner, "Open-Source Cancer Research," TED, October 2011, accessed September 27, 2013, http://www.ted.com/talks/jay_bradner_open_source_cancer_research.html.

17. Benjamin L. Ranard et al., "Crowdsourcing—Harnessing the Masses to Advance Health and Medicine, a Systematic Review," *Journal of General Internal Medicine* 29, no. 1 (2014): 187–203, doi: 10.1007/s11606-013-2536-8.

18. Amy Goldstein, telephone interview with author, Austin, Texas, October 7, 2013.

19. Occupational Safety and Health Administration, Department of Labor, "Hearing on Ergonomics," Stanford University, Palo Alto, California, July 24, 2001.

20. Kathryn Kobe, "Small Business GDP: Update 2002–2010," SBA.gov, January 2012, accessed January 20, 2014, http://www.sba.gov/sites/default/files/rs390tot_1.pdf.

21. Los Angeles Repetitive Strain Injury Support Group, "Report of the Workers' Compensation Reform Subcommittee: Recommendations on Workers' Compensation Reform," July 28, 2003.

9. TEENS AND TEXTING

1. Dino Drudi, "Brief: Have Disorders Associated with Repeated Trauma Stopped Increasing?" Bureau of Labor Statistics, Compensation and Working Conditions, summer 1997, accessed January 20, 2014, http://www.bls.gov/opub/mlr/cwc/have-disorders-associated-with-repeated-trauma-stopped-increasing.pdf.

2. Victoria J. Rideout, Ulla G. Foehr, and Donald F. Roberts, "Generation M2: Media in the Lives of 8 to 18 Year Olds," Kaiser Family Foundation, January 2010, accessed January 20, 2014, http://files.eric.ed.gov/fulltext/ED527859.pdf.

3. Rideout, Foehr, and Roberts, "Generation M2."

4. Rideout, Foehr, and Roberts, "Generation M2."

5. Liberty Mutual Research Institute for Safety, "Office Worker Safety: Ergonomic Interventions," *From Research to Reality* 15, no. 1 (summer 2012).

6. Jeff Teideman, loss-prevention specialist, telephone interview with author, Austin, Texas, October 6, 2013.

7. Judith Gold, Skype interview with author, Austin, Texas, July 30, 2013.

8. Isaiah W. Williams and Byron S. Kennedy, "Texting Tendonitis in a Teenager," *Journal of Family Practice* 60, no. 2 (February 2011): 66–67.

9. Gold, Skype interview.

10. Joseph J. Biundo, MD, and Perry J. Rush, MD, "Carpal Tunnel Syndrome," American College of Rheumatology, updated September 2012, accessed October 11, 2013, http://www.rheumatology.org/Practice/Clinical/Patients/Diseases_And_Conditions/Carpal_Tunnel_Syndrome.

11. Fred Steingold, "Repetitive Stress Injuries in the Workplace: Employers Should Use Workplace Ergonomics to Help Reduce Repetitive Stress Injuries on the Job," NOLO, accessed October 11, 2013, www.nolo.com/legal-encyclopedia/repetitive-stress-injuries-workplace-32281.html.

12. "CWCI Scorecard Looks at Carpal Tunnel Claims in California WC," WorkCompWire, January 11, 2013, accessed October 13, 2013, http://www.workcompwire.com/2013/01/cwci-scorecard-looks-at-carpal-tunnel-claims-in-california-wc.

13. Bonnie Prestridge, telephone interview with author, Austin, Texas, January 20, 2013.

14. Prestridge, telephone interview.

15. Bonnie Prestridge, Skype interview with author, Austin, Texas, October 14, 2013.

16. Steven Bryan, "Many Young People Suffer from 'Teen Texting Tendonitis': Sending Thousands of Text Messages per Month Can Lead to Back, Neck and Thumb Soreness," Yahoo! Voices, July 22, 2009, http://voices.yahoo.com/many-young-people-suffer-teen-texting-tendonitis-3862872.html?cat=15.

17. Greg Dempster, telephone interview with author, Austin, Texas, August 8, 2013.

18. Teideman, telephone interview.

19. "The Americans with Disabilities Act: A Primer for Small Business," US Equal Opportunity Employment Commission, http://www.eeoc.gov/eeoc/publications/adahandbook.cfm.

20. Small Business Administration, Office of Advocacy,http://www.sba.gov/advo.

21. Gold, Skype interview.

22. Paul Graham, "The Acceleration of Addictiveness," Paulgraham.com, July 2010, accessed October 15, 2013, http://paulgraham.com/addiction.html.

23. "Teaching with Documents: Photographs of Lewis Hine: Documentation of Child Labor," National Archives, http://www.archives.gov/education/lessons/hine-photos.

24. James U. McNeal, *Children as Consumers: Insights and Implications* (Lexington, MA: Lexington Books, 1986).

25. John Consoli, "Nickelodeon Study Affirms Kids' Strong Influence on Family Purchasing Decisions," Broadcasting and Cable, August 22, 2012, http://www.broadcastingcable.com/article/488764-Nickelodeon_Study_Affirms_Kids_Strong_Influence_on_Family_Purchasing_Decisions.php.

26. Consoli, "Nickelodeon Study Affirms Kids' Strong Influence on Family Purchasing Decisions."

10. EMPLOYERS AND RSIS

1. Eric J. Conn, "OSHA Launches Ergonomics Campaign in Healthcare Industries," Epstein Becker Green, August 12, 2013, accessed January 20, 2014, http://www.oshalawupdate.com/2013/08/12/osha-launches-ergonomics-campaign-in-healthcare-industries.

2. Small Business Administration, Office of Advocacy, http://www.sba.gov/advo.

3. Sheryll Poe, "The New Lawsuit Nightmares." FreeEnterprise.com, October 1, 2013, accessed January 20, 2014, www.freeenterprise.com/legal-reform/new-lawsuit-nightmares.

4. Jeff Teideman, loss-prevention specialist, telephone interview with author, Austin, Texas, October 6, 2013.

5. Sebastian Gonzales, "Active Release Techniques and OSHA," P2 Sports Care, accessed January 20, 2014, http://www.p2sportscare.com/preventative-care/active-release-technique-ocsa.

6. Mary Betsch, "One Company's Solution for Solving Strain/Sprain Injuries," *Leader 2004*, May 5, 2008, http://www.artcorpsolutions.com/services/on-site-wellness-prevention-programs.

7. Greg Dempster, Skype interview with author, Austin, Texas, October 3, 2013.

8. Judith Gold, Skype interview with author, Austin, Texas, July 30, 2013.

9. Robert Karasek and Tores Theorell, *Healthy Work: Stress, Productivity, and the Reconstruction of Working Life* (New York: Basic Books, 1992).

10. Steven Sauter et al., "Stress . . . at Work," Centers for Disease Control, DHHS (NIOSH) Publication Number 99-101, 1999, accessed January 20, 2014, http://www.cdc.gov/niosh/docs/99-101.

11. Liberty Mutual Research Institute for Safety, "Office Worker Safety: Ergonomic Interventions," *From Research to Reality* 15, no. 1 (summer 2012).

11. WHY RSIS COST YOU, EVEN IF YOU DON'T HAVE ONE

1. Mary Reaston, "Repetitive Stress Injury Has Become Cumulative Trauma for Employers," Insurance Thought Leadership, accessed October 21, 2013, http://www.insurancethoughtleadership.com/articles/repetitive-stress-injury-has-become-cumulative-trauma-for-employers#axzz2iOmTiRXa.

2. Jonny Evans, "Repetitive Strain Injury Costing Businesses Millions," Techworld.com, June, 5, 2008, http://www.techworld.com.au/article/223422/repetitive_strain_injury_costing_businesses_millions.

3. Jeremiah A. Barondess, MD, "Musculoskeletal Disorders in the Workplace: Low Back and Upper Extremities," National Academy of Sciences, April 26, 2001, accessed January 20, 2014, http://www7.nationalacademies.org/ocga/testimony/Musculoskeletal_Disorders_and_the_Workplace.asp.

4. Cathy Stanton, telephone interview with author, Austin, Texas, September 27, 2013.

5. Joseph LaDou, "Workers' Compensation in the United States: Cost Shifting and Inequities in a Dysfunctional System," *New Solutions* 20, no. 3 (2010): 291–302, http://workerscomphub.org/sites/default/files/resource-files/Workers'%20Compensation%20in%20the%20United%20States%20Cost%20Shifting%20and%20Inequities%20in%20a%20Dysfunctional%20System.pdf.

6. LaDou, "Workers' Compensation in the United States."

7. Z. J. Fan et al., "Underreporting of Work-Related Injury or Illness to Workers' Compensation: Individual and Industry Factors," *Journal of Occupational and Environmental Medicine* 48, no. 9 (2006): 914–22.

8. John Holahan, Dawn M. Miller, and David Rousseau, "Dual Eligibles: Medicaid Enrollment and Spending for Medicare Beneficiaries in 2005," Kaiser Commission, Publication 7846, February 2009, http://www.kff.org/medicaid/7846.cfm; G. F. Riley, "The Cost of Eliminating the 24-Month Medicare Waiting Period for Social Security Disabled-Worker Beneficiaries," *Medical Care* 42, no. 4 (2004): 387–94.

9. Richard Finger, "Fraud and Disability Equal a Multibillion Dollar Black Hole for Taxpayers," *Forbes*, October 19, 2013, http://www.forbes.com/sites/richardfinger/2013/01/14/fraud-and-disability-equal-a-multibillion-dollar-balck-hole-for-taxpayers.

10. Finger, "Fraud and Disability."

11. "Investigative Report Reveals Disability Costs Twice as Much as Welfare, Food Stamps Combined," Catholic Online, March 26, 2013, http://www.catholic.org/politics/story.php?id=50272#.UmGmz7IepE8.email.

12. Finger, "Fraud and Disability."

13. "Investigative Report Reveals Disability Costs Twice as Much as Welfare, Food Stamps Combined."

14. LaDou, "Workers' Compensation in the United States."

15. Finger, "Fraud and Disability."

16. Finger, "Fraud and Disability."

17. David G. Allen, PhD, SPHR, "Retaining Talent," Society for Human Resource Management, 2008, accessed January 18, 2014, http://www.shrm.org/about/foundation/research/documents/retaining%20talent-%20final.pdf.

18. Adrian Wooldridge, "The Battle for Brainpower," *Economist*, October 5, 2006, accessed January 20, 2014, http://www.economist.com/node/7961894.

19. Kevin A. Hassett and Robert J. Shapiro, "What Ideas Are Worth: The Value of Intellectual Capital and Intangible Assets in the American Economy." Sonecon, October 2011, accessed January 20, 2014, http://www.sonecon.com/docs/studies/Value_of_Intellectual_Capital_in_American_Economy.pdf.

20. W. F. Cascio, *Managing Human Resources: Productivity, Quality of Work Life, Profits*, 7th ed. (Burr Ridge, IL: Irwin/McGraw-Hill, 2006); Terence R. Mitchell et al., "How to Keep Your Best Employees: Developing an Effective Retention Policy," *Academy of Management Executive* 15 (2001): 96–108.

21. Cascio, *Managing Human Resources*.

22. Saveri Hammonds, "Can Ernst and Young Retain Women by Rethinking Work?" *Businessweek*, February 23, 1998.

23. "Confronting the Talent Crunch: 2008," A Manpower Whitepaper, Experis Manpower-Group, 2008, accessed January 21, 2014, https://candidate.manpower.com/wps/wcm/connect/SGCampus/1d21eb804ec2f611baa3fbee16aecd97/TalentCrunch2008_USLetter.pdf?MOD=AJPERES.

12. WHY WORK IS THE CURE FOR RSIS

1. Fritjof Capra, *The Turning Point: Science, Society, and the Rising Culture* (New York: Bantam, 1984).

2. Robert Karasek and Tores Theorell, *Healthy Work: Stress, Productivity, and the Reconstruction of Working Life* (New York: Basic Books, 1992).

3. Karasek and Theorell, *Healthy Work*.

4. J. W. M. Kessels, "What Is beyond Knowledge Productivity?" In *Beyond Knowledge Productivity: Report of a Quest*, edited by T. van Aken and T. M. van Engers, 19–28. Utrecht: LEMMA, 1996.

5. "Stress at Work." MedicineNet, www.medicinenet.com/health_and_the_workplace/article.htm.

6. Jeff Teideman, telephone interview with author, Austin, Texas, October 6, 2013.

7. Judith Gold, Skype interview with author, Austin, Texas, July 30, 2013.

8. Steve Jex and Thomas Britt, *Organizational Psychology: A Scientist-Practitioner Approach*, 2nd ed. (New York: Wiley, 2008).

9. Bonnie Prestridge, Skype interview with author, Austin, Texas, October 15, 2013.

10. Prestridge, Skype interview.

11. Prestridge, Skype interview.

12. Matthew Fox, *The Reinvention of Work* (San Francisco: Harper, 1994), 5.

13. Prestridge, Skype interview.

Bibliography

Allen, David G., PhD, SPHR. "Retaining Talent." Society for Human Resource Management, 2008, accessed January 18, 2014, http://www.shrm.org/about/foundation/research/documents/retaining%20talent-%20final.pdf.

American Academy of Orthopaedic Surgeons (AAOS). "AAOS Clinical Guidelines on the Treatment of Carpal Tunnel Syndrome." *AAOS Now*, October 2008, accessed February 6, 2014, http://www.aaos.org/news/aaosnow/oct08/clinical3.asp.

"The Americans with Disabilities Act: A Primer for Small Business." US Equal Opportunity Employment Commission, accessed February 6, 2014, http://www.eeoc.gov/eeoc/publications/adahandbook.cfm.

Atwood, Shelly, cardiopulmonary specialist and filmmaker. Telephone interview with author. Austin, Texas, September 15, 2013.

Bailin, Jonathan, ergonomist. Telephone interview with author. Austin, Texas, June 14, 2013.

Ball, Christopher A. *Take Charge of Your Workers' Compensation Claim: An A to Z Guide for Injured Employees*. 2nd ed. Berkeley, CA: Nolo, 2001.

Bammer, Gabriele, and Brian Martin. "Repetition Strain Injury in Australia: Medical Knowledge, Social Movement, and De Facto Partisanship." *Social Problems* 39, no. 3 (August 1992): 219–37.

Barondess, Jeremiah A., MD. "Muscoloskeletal Disorders in the Workplace: Low Back and Upper Extremities." National Academy of Sciences, April 26, 2001, accessed January 20, 2014, http://www7.nationalacademies.org/ocga/testimony/Musculoskeletal_Disorders_and_the_Workplace.asp.

Bellamy, Paul B. *A History of Workmen's Compensation, 1898–1915: From Courtroom to Boardroom*. New York and London: Garland Publishing, 1997.

Berzon, Alexandra, and Melanie Trottman. "OSHA Seeks to Make Injury Records Public." *Wall Street Journal*, November 7, 2013, accessed February 6, 2014, http://online.wsj.com/news/articles/SB10001424052702304672404579182480900278574.

Betsch, Mary. "One Company's Solution for Solving Strain/Sprain Injuries." *Leader 2004*, May 5, 2008, accessed February 6, 2014, http://www.artcorpsolutions.com/services/on-site-wellness-prevention-programs.

Biundo, Joseph J., MD, and Perry J. Rush, MD. "Carpal Tunnel Syndrome." American College of Rheumatology, updated September 2012, accessed October 11, 2013, http://www.rheumatology.org/Practice/Clinical/Patients/Diseases_And_Conditions/Carpal_Tunnel_Syndrome.

Bradner, Jay. "Open-Source Cancer Research." TED, October 2011, accessed September 27, 2013, http://www.ted.com/talks/jay_bradner_open_source_cancer_research.html.

Bryan, Steven. "Many Young People Suffer from 'Teen Texting Tendonitis': Sending Thousands of Text Messages per Month Can Lead to Back, Neck and Thumb Soreness." Yahoo! Voices, July 22, 2009, accessed February 6, 2014, http://voices.yahoo.com/many-young-people-suffer-teen-texting-tendonitis-3862872.html?cat=15.

Bush, Lamar, board-certified bodyworker. In-person interview with author. Austin, Texas, June 3, 2013.

California Commission on Health and Safety and Workers' Compensation. *2012 Annual Report*. State of California, Labor and Workforce Development Agency, Department of Industrial Relations, December 2012.

Capra, Fritjof. *The Turning Point: Science, Society, and the Rising Culture*. New York: Bantam, 1984.

"Carpal Tunnel Syndrome." *New York Times*, February 17, 2011, accessed May 26, 2012, http://health.nytimes.com/health/guides/disease/carpal-tunnel-syndrome/prognosis.html.

Cascio, W. F. *Managing Human Resources: Productivity, Quality of Work Life, Profits*. 7th ed. Burr Ridge, IL: Irwin/McGraw-Hill, 2006.

Claussen, Lauretta. "Workplace Myth? Carpal Tunnel Syndrome from Computer Use Unlikely, Experts Claim." *Safety and Health Magazine*, October 1, 2011, accessed November 18, 2013, http://www.safetyandhealthmagazine.com/articles/6383-workplace-myth.

Collins, James D., MD, radiologist. Telephone interview with author. Austin, Texas, August 5, 2013.

"Computer Usage in the U.S." Pew Internet and American Life Project Tracking Survey, December 2008, accessed May 26, 2012, http://www.infoplease.com/ipa/A0921872.html#ixzz1w0G4V2I5.

"Confronting the Talent Crunch: 2008," A Manpower Whitepaper, Experis ManpowerGroup, 2008, accessed January 21, 2014, https://candidate.manpower.com/wps/wcm/connect/SGCampus/1d21eb804ec2f611baa3fbee16aecd97/TalentCrunch2008_USLetter.pdf?MOD=AJPERES.

Conn, Eric J. "OSHA Launches Ergonomics Campaign in Healthcare Industries." Epstein Becker Green, August 12, 2013, accessed January 20, 2014, http://www.oshalawupdate.com/2013/08/12/osha-launches-ergonomics-campaign-in-healthcare-industries.

Consoli, John. "Nickelodeon Study Affirms Kids' Strong Influence on Family Purchasing Decisions." *Broadcasting and Cable*, August 22, 2012, http://www.broadcastingcable.com/article/488764-Nickelodeon_Study_Affirms_Kids_Strong_Influence_on_Family_Purchasing_Decisions.php.

"The Cost of Work-Related Injury and Illness for Australian Employers, Workers and the Community 2008–09." Safe Work Australia, 2012, accessed February 6, 2014, http://www.safeworkaustralia.gov.au/sites/swa/about/publications/pages/cost-injury-illness-2008-09.

Cowan, Penney, founder of the Chronic Pain Association. Telephone interview with author. Austin, Texas, July 2, 2013.

Cuddy, Ann. "Your Body Language Shapes Who You Are." TED, October 2012, accessed October 1, 2013, http://www.ted.com/talks/amy_cuddy_your_body_language_shapes_who_you_are.html.

Cuomo, Andrew M. "Governor Cuomo Details Improvements to New York's Workers' Compensation System That Cut Costs to Employers by 26% for 2014," Office of the Governor, Albany, New York, October 30, 2013, accessed February 6, 2014, https://www.governor.ny.gov/press/10302013-ny-workers-compensation-system.

"CWCI Scorecard Looks at Carpal Tunnel Claims in California WC." WorkCompWire, January 11, 2013, accessed October 13, 2013, http://www.workcompwire.com/2013/01/cwci-scorecard-looks-at-carpal-tunnel-claims-in-california-wc.

Daley, Adam. "CDC Survey: Carpal Tunnel Syndrome Mostly Linked to Work." MedicalDaily.com, December 23, 2011, accessed October 13, 2013, http://www.medicaldaily.com/cdc-survey-carpal-tunnel-syndrome-mostly-linked-work-239127.

DeBecker, Gavin. *The Gift of Fear: Survival Signals That Protect Us from Violence*. Boston: Little, Brown, 1997.

Dempster, Greg, ergonomist. Telephone interview with author. Austin, Texas, August 8, 2013.
———. Skype interview with author. Austin, Texas, October 3, 2013.

Dickerson, Marla. "Chiropractic Claims Pain California Employers." *Los Angeles Times*, August 17, 2003, accessed October 27, 2013, http://articles.latimes.com/2003/aug/17/business/fi-chiro17.

Dixon, Lloyd, James W. Macdonald, and William Barbagallo. "California's Volatile Workers' Compensation Insurance Market: Problems and Recommendations for Change." Prepared for the Commission on Health and Safety and Workers' Compensation, Rand Corporation, Center for Health and Safety in the Workplace and Navigant Consulting, 2009, accessed February 6, 2014, http://www.dir.ca.gov/chswc/reports/2009/insolvencyreport.pdf.

Dougherty, Paul. "Public Health, Musculoskeletal Disorders and Chiropractic: The Time Is Now." American Public Health Association, fall 2009, accessed May 26, 2012, http://www.apha.org/membergroups/newsletters/sectionnewsletters/chiro/fall09/doughtery.htm.

Drudi, Dino. "Brief: Have Disorders Associated with Repeated Trauma Stopped Increasing?" Bureau of Labor Statistics, Compensation and Working Conditions, summer 1997, accessed January 20, 2014, www.bls.gov/opub/mlr/cwc/have-disorders-associated-with-repeated-trauma-stopped-increasing.pdf.

Edgelow, Peter I., PT. "A New Perspective on the Etiology, Evaluation and Management of Patients with Signs and Symptoms of Chronic Pain and Cumulative Trauma Disorder." Presented at the Los Angeles Repetitive Strain Injury Support Group, Wellspring Therapy Clinic, Glendale, California, October 2000.

"Employer and Insurer Fraud: Boosting Bottom Line Profits at the Expense of Workers and Society." Workers Injury Law and Advocacy Group, October 2011.

Evans, Jonny. "Repetitive Strain Injury Costing Businesses Millions." Techworld.com, June 5, 2008, accessed February 6, 2014, http://www.techworld.com.au/article/223422/repetitive_strain_injury_costing_businesses_millions.

Fan, Z. J., D. K. Bonauto, M. P. Foley, and B.A. Silverstein. "Underreporting of Work-Related Injury or Illness to Workers' Compensation: Individual and Industry Factors." *Journal of Occupational and Environmental Medicine* 48, no. 9 (2006): 914–22.

Finger, Richard. "Fraud and Disability Equal a Multibillion Dollar Black Hole for Taxpayers." *Forbes*, October 19, 2013, accessed February 6, 2014, http://www.forbes.com/sites/richardfinger/2013/01/14/fraud-and-disability-equal-a-multibillion-dollar-balck-hole-for-taxpayers.

Foley, Greg. "Occupational Health and Safety in Australian Workplaces—the High Risk and High Cost of Serious Body Stressing Incidents," National and Workplace Statistics and Epidemiology Team, National Occupational Health and Safety Commission, November 1996.

Fox, Matthew. *The Reinvention of Work*. San Francisco: Harper, 1994.

Garfinkel, Marian S., EdD, adjunct professor, Temple University Medical School, Senior Level III Iyengar yoga instructor. Telephone interview with author. Austin, Texas, September 9, 2013.

Garfinkel, Marian S., Atul Singhal, Warren A. Katz, David A. Allan, Rosemary Reshetar, and H. Ralph Schumacher Jr. "Yoga-Based Intervention for Carpal Tunnel Syndrome: A Randomized Trial." *JAMA* 280, no. 18 (1998): 1601–3, doi: 10.1001/jama.280.18.1601.

Gawande, Atul. "How Do We Heal Medicine?" TED, April 2012, accessed August 18, 2013, http://www.ted.com/talks/atul_gawande_how_do_we_heal_medicine.html.

Gold, Judith, ergonomist and epidemiologist. Skype interview with author. Austin, Texas, July 30, 2013.

Goldstein, Amy, State Pain Policy Advocacy Network. Telephone interview with author. Austin, Texas, October 7, 2013.

Gonzales, Sebastian. "Active Release Techniques and OSHA." P2 Sports Care, accessed January 20, 2014, http://www.p2sportscare.com/preventative-care/active-release-technique-ocsa.

Graham, Paul. "The Acceleration of Addictiveness." Paulgraham.com, July 2010, accessed October 15, 2013, http://paulgraham.com/addiction.html.

Hammonds, Saveri. "Can Ernst and Young Retain Women by Rethinking Work?" *Businessweek*, February 23, 1998.

Hardberger, Phil. "Texas Workers' Compensation: A Ten Year Survey—Strengths, Weaknesses, and Recommendations." 32 St. Mary's L.J. 1, 6 (2000).

Hassett, Kevin A., and Robert J. Shapiro. "What Ideas Are Worth: The Value of Intellectual Capital and Intangible Assets in the American Economy." Sonecon, October 2011, accessed January 20, 2014, http://www.sonecon.com/docs/studies/Value_of_Intellectual_Capital_in_American_Economy.pdf.

Healey, Bernard J., and Kenneth T. Walker. *Introduction to Occupational Health in Public Health Practice.* New York: Wiley and Sons, 2009.

Heussner, Ki Mae. "Teen Gets Carpal Tunnel from Texting." ABC News, March 19, 2010, accessed September 19, 2013, http://abcnews.go.com/Technology/teen-carpal-tunnel-texting/story?id=10146773.

Holahan, John, Dawn M. Miller, and David Rousseau. "Dual Eligibles: Medicaid Enrollment and Spending for Medicare Beneficiaries in 2005." Kaiser Commission, Publication 7846, February 2009, accessed February 6, 2014, http://www.kff.org/medicaid/7846.cfm.

Ibrahim, I., W. S. Khan, N. Goddard, and P. Smitham. "Carpal Tunnel Syndrome: A Review of the Recent Literature," *Open Orthopaedics Journal* 6 (2012): 69–76.

In re J. D. Edwards World Solutions Co., 87 S.W.3d 546 at 549 (Tex. 2002).

"Investigative Report Reveals Disability Costs Twice as Much as Welfare, Food Stamps Combined." Catholic Online, March 26, 2013, accessed September 26, 2013, http://www.catholic.org/politics/story.php?id=50272#.UmGmz7IepE8.email.

Jergler, Don. "Carriers 'Uncertain' about California Workers' Comp Reform." *Insurance Journal*, December 19, 2012, accessed August 23, 2013, http://www.insurancejournal.com/news/west/2012/12/19/274774.htm.

Jex, Steve, and Thomas Britt. *Organizational Psychology: A Scientist-Practitioner Approach.* 2nd ed. New York: Wiley, 2008.

Juhan, Deane. *Job's Body: A Handbook for Bodywork.* Barrytown, NY: Barrytown, 1998.

Kanji, Giresh. "The Flight/Fight Response in Chronic Pain." Southern Cross Hospital, accessed February 6, 2014, http://sportsandpain.co.nz/painclinic/wp-content/uploads/2012/04/Advice-sheet-adrenaline.pdf.

Karasek, Robert and Tores Theorell. *Healthy Work: Stress, Productivity, and the Reconstruction of Working Life.* New York: Basic Books, 1992.

Kessels, J. W. M. "What Is beyond Knowledge Productivity?" In *Beyond Knowledge Productivity: Report of a Quest*, edited by T. van Aken and T. M. van Engers, 19–28. Utrecht: LEMMA, 1996.

Kobe, Kathryn. "Small Business GDP: Update 2002–2010." SBA.gov, January 2012, accessed January 20, 2014, http://www.sba.gov/sites/default/files/rs390tot_1.pdf.

LaDou, Joseph. "Workers' Compensation in the United States: Cost Shifting and Inequities in a Dysfunctional System." *New Solutions* 20, no. 3 (2010): 291–302, http://workerscomphub.org/sites/default/files/resource-files/.

Lenhart, Amanda. "Teens, Smartphones & Texting." Pew Research Center's Internet and American Life Project, March 19, 2012, accessed January 20, 2014, http://www.pewinternet.org/~/media/Files/Reports/2012/PIP_Teens_Smartphones_and_Texting.pdf.

Liberty Mutual Research Institute for Safety. "Office Worker Safety: Ergonomic Interventions." *From Research to Reality* 15, no. 1 (summer 2012).

Lockhart, R. D., G. F. Hamilton, and F. W. Fyfe. *Anatomy of the Human Body.* Philadelphia: J. B. Lippincott, 1965.

López-Alonso, Mónica, Rosalía Pacheco Torres, Eulalia Jadraque Gago, and Javier Ordoñez García. "The Health Effects of Vibrations on the Upper Extremities of Workers." Prepared for the Global Virtual Conference, University of Granada, Department of Projects and Construction Engineering, April 8–12, 2013.

Los Angeles Repetitive Strain Injury Support Group. "Report of the Workers' Compensation Reform Subcommittee: Recommendations on Workers' Compensation Reform," July 28, 2003.

Luckhaupt, S. E., J. M. Dahlhamer, B. W. Ward, M. H. Sweeney, J. P. Sestito, and G. M. Calvert. "Prevalence and Work-Relatedness of Carpal Tunnel Syndrome in the Working Population." 2010 National Health Interview Survey. *American Journal of Industrial Medicine*, accessed May 26, 2012, doi: 10.1002/ajim.22048.

Mandel, Peter, MD. Comment made at US Department of Labor, Public Forums on Ergonomics, Stanford University, California, July 24, 2001.

McNeal, James U. *Children as Consumers: Insights and Implications*. Lexington, MA: Lexington Books, 1986.

Mitchell, Terence R., Brooks C. Holtom, Thomas W. Lee, and Ted Graske. "How to Keep Your Best Employees: Developing an Effective Retention Policy." *Academy of Management Executive* 15 (2001): 96–108.

"National OHS Strategy 2002–2012: Priority Mechanism Progress." Safe Work Australia, 2012, accessed February 6, 2014, http://www.safeworkaustralia.gov.au/sites/SWA/about/Publications/Documents/232/, chapter 8, note 14.

"New Jersey Spine and Rehabilitation," last modified 2012, accessed February 6, 2014, http://askthetrucker.com/increase-in-spinal-back-pain-among-long-haul-truck-drivers.

New York State Workers' Compensation Board. *New York Carpal Tunnel Syndrome Medical Treatment Guidelines*. New York: New York Workers' State Compensation Board, 2013.

"Occupational Overuse Syndrome." XTRA: Health: A–Z of Health, January 3, 2001, accessed October 8, 2001, http://222.xtra.co.nz/health/0,,747-38487,00.html.

Occupational Safety and Health Administration. "Enforcement." OSHA, accessed September 25, 2013, https://www.osha.gov/SLTC/ergonomics/faqs.html.

Occupational Safety and Health Administration, Department of Labor. "Hearing on Ergonomics." Stanford University, Palo Alto, California, July 24, 2001.

Pascarelli, Emil, and Deborah Quilter. *Repetitive Strain Injury: A Computer User's Guide*. New York: Wiley, 1994.

Pear, Robert. "Percentage of Americans Lacking Health Coverage Falls Again." *New York Times*, September 17, 2013, accessed October 1, 2013, http://www.nytimes.com/2013/09/18/us/percentage-of-americans-lacking-health-coverage-falls-again.html?_r=0.

Pereira, W., P. Tittiranonda, and S. Burastero. "Ergonomic Analysis of Movement Retraining of Computer Users: A Pilot Study." Presented at the Triennial IEA/HFES Conference, San Diego, California, August 2000.

Piligian, George J., MD. Telephone interview with author. Austin, Texas, August 11, 2013.

Poe, Sheryll. "The New Lawsuit Nightmares." FreeEnterprise.com, October 1, 2013, accessed January 20, 2014, http://www.freeenterprise.com/legal-reform/new-lawsuit-nightmares.

Prestridge, Bonnie, RSI sufferer. Telephone and Skype interviews with author. Austin, Texas, January 20, 2013, and October 14, 2013.

Purcell, Kristen. "E-Reader Ownership Doubles in Six Months." Pew Internet Project, June 27, 2011, accessed May 26, 2012, http://pewInternet.org/~/media/Files/Reports/2011/PIP_eReader_Tablet.pdf.

Ranard, Benjamin L., Yoonhee P. Ha, Zach F. Meisel, David A. Asch, Shawndra Hill, Lance B. Becker, Anne K. Seymour, and Raina M. Merchant. "Crowdsourcing—Harnessing the Masses to Advance Health and Medicine, a Systematic Review." *Journal of General Internal Medicine* 29, no. 1 (2014): 187–203, doi: 10.1007/s11606-013-2536-8.

Reaston, Mary. "Repetitive Stress Injury Has Become Cumulative Trauma for Employers." Insurance Thought Leadership, accessed October 21, 2013, http://www.insurancethoughtleadership.com/articles/repetitive-stress-injury-has-become-cumulative-trauma-for-employers#axzz2iOmTiRXa.

Rideout, Victoria J., Ulla G. Foehr, and Donald F. Roberts. "Generation M2: Media in the Lives of 8 to 18 Year Olds." Kaiser Family Foundation, January 2010, accessed January 20, 2014,http://files.eric.ed.gov/fulltext/ED527859.pdf.

Riley, G. F. "The Cost of Eliminating the 24-Month Medicare Waiting Period for Social Security Disabled-Worker Beneficiaries." *Medical Care* 42, no. 4 (2004): 387–94, accessed February 4, 2014, http://www.ssa.gov/policy/docs/ssb/v52n5/v52n5p2.pdf.

Rohrlich, Ted, and Evelyn Larrubia. "Public Fraud Unit Favors Those Who Privately Fund It." *Los Angeles Times*, August 6, 2000, accessed February 6, 2014, http://articles.latimes.com/2000/aug/06/news/mn-65499.

RSI and Overuse Injury Association of the Act, Inc. Newsletter. ACT Health and the Southern Cross Club, autumn 2013.

Sauter, Steven, Lawrence Murphy, Michael Colligan, Naomi Swanson, Joseph Hurrell Jr., Frederick Scharf Jr., Raymond Sinclair, Paula Grubb, Linda Goldenhar, Toni Alterman, Janet Johnston, Anne Hamilton, and Julie Tisdale. "Stress . . . at Work." Centers for Disease Control, DHHS (NIOSH) Publication Number 99-101, 1999, accessed January 20, 2014, http://www.cdc.gov/niosh/docs/99-101.

Schiottz-Christensen, Berit, Vert Mooney, Shadi Azad, Dan Selstad, Jennifer Gulick, and Mark Bracker. "The Role of Active Release Manual Therapy for Upper Extremity Overuse Syndromes—a Preliminary Report." *Journal of Occupational Rehabilitation* 9, no. 3 (September 1999): 201–11.

Sengupta, Ishita, Marjorie Baldwin, and Virginia Reno. *Workers' Compensation: Benefits, Coverage, and Costs, 2011.* National Academy of Social Insurance, August 2013, accessed January 20, 2014, http://www.nasi.org/research/2013/report-workers-compensation-benefits-coverage-costs-2011.

Sims, N. R., and H. Muyderman. "Mitochondria, Oxidative Metabolism and Cell Death in Stroke." *Biochimica et Biophysica Acta* 1802, no. 1 (January 2010): 80–91.

Smith, Aaron. "35 Percent of American Adults Own a Smartphone." Pew Internet Project, July 11, 2011, accessed May 26, 2012, http://pewInternet.org/~/media//Files/Reports/2011/PIP_Smartphones.pdf.

———. "Mobile Access 2010." Pew Internet Project, July 7, 2010, accessed May 26, 2012, http://www.pewInternet.org/~/media/Files/Reports/2010/PIP_Mobile_Access_2010.pdf.

Smith, Steve, Richard Gannon, and Peggy Sugarman. *Annual Report for 1998.* California Department of Industrial Relations, Division of Workers' Compensation, accessed April 1, 2002, http://www.dir.ca.gov/DWC/98DWCAR.htm.

Sommer, Roger D. "Retaining Intellectual Capital in the 21st Century." OI Partners, January 13, 2011, http://aka-oi.com/newsroom/newsletter/jan-2011-newsletter/11-01-13/Retaining_Intellectual_Capital_in_the_21st_Century.aspx.

Spognardi, Mark A., and Staci L. Ketay. "Perspective—Bad Law and Bad Politics: OSHA's Ill-Fated Ergonomics Standard." *Employee Relations Law Journal* 27, no. 1 (summer 2001): 85–90.

Station, Cathy, attorney. Telephone interview with author. Austin, Texas, September 27, 2013.

Steingold, Fred. "Repetitive Stress Injuries in the Workplace: Employers Should Use Workplace Ergonomics to Help Reduce Repetitive Stress Injuries on the Job." NOLO, accessed October 11, 2013, http://www.nolo.com/legal-encyclopedia/repetitive-stress-injuries-workplace-32281.html.

Stewart, R. S., M. D. Devous Sr., A. J. Rush, L. Lane, and F. J. Bonte. "Cerebral Blood Flow Changes during Sodium-Lactate-Induced Panic Attacks." *American Journal of Psychiatry* 145, no. 4 (April 1988): 442–49.

Stewart, Walter F., Judith A. Ricci, Elsbeth Chee, David Morganstein, and Richard Lipton. "Lost Productive Time and Cost Due to Common Pain Conditions in the US Workforce." *JAMA* 290, no. 18 (2003): 2443–54, accessed May 27, 2012, doi: 10.1001/jama.290.18.2443.

"Stress at Work." MedicineNet, accessed October 11, 2013, http://www.medicinenet.com/health_and_the_workplace/article.htm.

Tang, N. K. Y., and C. Crane. "Suicidality in Chronic Pain: A Review of the Prevalence, Risk Factors and Psychological Links." *Psychological Medicine* 36 (2006): 575–86, doi: 10.1017/S0033291705006859.

"Teaching with Documents: Photographs of Lewis Hine: Documentation of Child Labor." National Archives, accessed October 19, 2013, http://www.archives.gov/education/lessons/hine-photos.

Teideman, Jeff, loss-prevention specialist. Telephone interview with author. Austin, Texas, October 6, 2013.

Thornton, Gary A. "Walmart Opted Out, but the Sky Is Not Falling." *State Bar of Texas Workers' Compensation Section Newsletter* 1, no. 6 (summer 2012), accessed January 20, 2014, http://www.texasworkerscompensationsection.com/Newsletters/summer2012.pdf.

Washington Health Policy Fellows. "Musculoskeletal Education in Medical Schools: Are We Making the Cut?" American Association of Orthopaedic Surgeons, March–April 2007, http://www.aaos.org/news/bulletin/marapr07/reimbursement2.asp.

"What Is Ergonomics?" International Ergonomics Association, 2000, accessed January 20, 2014, http://www.iea.cc/whats/index.html.

Williams, David A., PhD. Telephone interview with author. Austin, Texas, July 9, 2013.

Williams, Isaiah W., and Byron S. Kennedy. "Texting Tendonitis in a Teenager." *Journal of Family Practice* 60, no. 2 (February 2011): 66–67.

Wooldridge, Adrian. "The Battle for Brainpower." *Economist*, October 5, 2006, accessed January 20, 2014, http://www.economist.com/node/7961894.

Index

About the Author

Jill Gambaro has lived with multiple repetitive strain injuries known as a "double crush" for over thirteen years. A former member of the board of directors of the Los Angeles Repetitive Strain Injury Support Group and the Cumulative Trauma Disorders Resource Network, Jill has interviewed hundreds of doctors, lawyers, physical therapists, alternative healers, injured workers, members of the workers' compensation community, and RSI sufferers. She has met with representatives from Senators Feinstein and Boxer's offices; wrote an article entitled "Is Work Killing Us?" for the *Washington Free Press*; spoke at the California state capitol during a press conference on the California Workers' Compensation System; appeared on *Which Way LA?* on National Public Radio's KCET station in Los Angeles; as well as KCAL-KCBS five o'clock and eleven o'clock news to discuss reforms in the California Workers' Compensation system. She is a professional writer and film producer. For more information visit: www.truthaboutcarpaltunnel.com.